THE NEW ILLUSTRATED

MEDICAL and HEALTH ENCYCLOPEDIA

Unified Edition

COMPLETE IN 18
VOLUMES

This 18 volume edition contains new entries, illustrations, anatomical charts and MEDIGRAPHS plus matter from THE MODERN HOME MEDICAL ADVISER and THE MODERN FAMILY HEALTH GUIDE.

VOLUME
2

ALOES
BATHING BABY

THE *New* ILLUSTRATED MEDICAL and HEALTH ENCYCLOPEDIA

EDITED BY

MORRIS FISHBEIN, M.D.

EDITOR, Medical Progress
EDITOR, Modern Home Medical Advisor
EDITOR, Excerpta Medica
CONTRIBUTING EDITOR, Postgraduate Medicine
MEDICAL EDITOR, Encyclopedia Book of the Year
FORMERLY EDITOR, Journal of the American Medical Association

With the Collaboration of 50 Leading Specialists in Medicine and Surgery

H. S. STUTTMAN CO., Inc. *Publishers*
New York, N.Y. 10016

UNIFIED EDITION
THE NEW ILLUSTRATED MEDICAL AND HEALTH ENCYCLOPEDIA

Library of Congress Catalog Card Number 7-125825

PRINTED IN THE UNITED STATES OF AMERICA

VOLUME 2

ALOES TO BATHING BABY

CONSULTING DISCUSSIONS

MEDIGRAPHS

COLOR PLATES, MEDICAL CHARTS, PHOTO FEATURES

ALOES, a brownish yellow powder, obtained from the dried juice of the leaves of the *aloe,* a plant found in the West Indies and Africa. Aloes is used in chronic constipation for its stimulating effect on the large intestine. Large doses taken too frequently may irritate the kidneys.

ALOPECIA, loss of hair that may follow a number of different illnesses. The loss of hair may be partial or total, premature or senile. If hair falls in patches, the condition is known as *alopecia areata. Alopecia cachectica* is baldness as a result of general malnutrition. *See also* BALDNESS.

ALTITUDE SICKNESS, a term given to any of several disorders which may develop in certain individuals at high altitudes to which they are unaccustomed. For example, such disorders may occur among visitors to the Andes mountains in South America, where many of the towns and cities are located at elevations of from 8,000 to 14,000 feet.

Symptoms include an increase in the rate and depth of breathing (in inverse proportion to the decrease of oxygen pressure), and an increase in the number of red blood cells and the amount of hemoglobin (the function of which is to carry oxygen to the cells of the body). Other symptoms include dizziness, inertia, headache, vomiting, difficulty in hearing and seeing, nosebleed, and —at very great heights—fever. There may also be weakness in the legs.

If efforts are made slowly, one gradually becomes accustomed to the higher altitude. For severe symptoms, administration of a mixture of pure oxygen with air gives relief.

Altitude sickness was formerly a problem in aviation. Today, most airplane compartments are pressurized, and this is no longer ordinarily the case. Of course, altitude sickness can still occur to individuals travelling in unpressurized airplanes at great heights.

Altitude sickness is likely to occur among mountain climbers, unless they bring along an ample supply of pure oxygen. At 18,000 feet, about 25 per cent of normal people collapse within a period of one-half to one hour unless they are provided with extra oxygen. Associated with this may be changes in mental function and emotional control which may result in disturbances of judgment. *See also* MOUNTAIN SICKNESS; MOTION SICKNESS; EAR STUFFINESS; SPACE MEDICINE.

► Home Care of Common Ailments, *Motion Sickness,* 1676.

ALUM, a crystalline substance, colorless and odorless, which dissolves in water; an effective emetic in cases of poisoning, but seldom given internally. Although alum is strongly astringent, its use as an after-shaving styptic is not recommended. Any of the packaged stringent surgical powders which can be used in small amounts as needed and applied directly to a bleeding point are preferable. *See also* POISONING.

ALUMINUM. When aluminum is taken into the body a small amount of the substance remains, chiefly in the liver and spleen. Most of the aluminum is promptly passed from the body in the urine and in the bile. The body easily takes care of any insignificant amounts of this metal that may be ingested as a result of eating food cooked in aluminum cooking utensils. There is no evidence that aluminum absorbed as a result of using aluminum cooking utensils has any harmful effect on the ordinary consumer. The claim has been made that aluminum in foods or the use of aluminum cooking utensils in some manner may promote the growth of cancer in the human body. There is not the slightest scientific evidence to support this claim.

Aluminum is used in medicine in the form of an *aluminum hydroxide gel* which is prescribed chiefly as an antacid substance in the treatment of ulcer of the stomach and duodenum or whenever there seems to be excessive acid in the stomach. It has a slight astringent effect and serves also to coat the affected area and thus to protect it against the action of acid. Furthermore, such gels of aluminum hydroxide tend to increase the mucin secretion, which is also favorable to the treatment of ulcer. Many different preparations of this type are now available and are frequently prescribed by physicians. They should not, of course, be taken unless prescribed by the doctor for the specific case and in the amounts which he thinks desirable in that case.

Another preparation of aluminum which is used in medicine is called *aluminum acetate.* This is used as a mild astringent and an antiseptic substance in dermatology. Many of the preparations used for sunburn and also those used to prevent underarm perspiration contain substances of this type.

Since the substance may be irritating in high concentration, it is customary for the doctor to prescribe it sufficiently diluted with water to make it harmless.

ALUMINUM ACETATE, an astringent used chiefly in a mild 5 per cent concentration in Burow's solution for wet dressings for minor skin disorders, boils, and in the treatment of *erysipelas.* It also brings relief in the initial stages of sunburn.

ALUMINUM HYDROXIDE, a white, gluelike substance used chiefly to neutralize stomach acidity. In the treatment of peptic ulcer it acts as a healing agent, relieving pain and controlling hemorrhage. When the liquid preparation is not tolerable, aluminum hydroxide may be obtained in gel or tablet form, which is the dried aluminum hydroxide gel. *See also* ANTACID; PEPTIC ULCER.

ALUMINUM PHOSPHATE GEL, an aluminum salt, similar in action and uses to aluminum hydroxide gel but preferable when milder drugs are desirable.

ALVEOLI, the small air cells of the lung, formed by terminal dilatations of the bronchioles.

AMAUROSIS, loss of vision due to nervous disorders and not to any structural defect of the eye.

AMBITION. The strong desire to gain position, recognition, or power is a form of self-seeking that is definitely a part of growing up. Ambition takes different forms, depending on the traditions and culture in which one lives, but also, for any individual child, depending upon his family—its status and means.

Children's early ambitions are largely determined by what they see others do, by what they hear praised or admired. It is natural for children to emulate their parents at one stage and the older boys and girls they come to know at another. They find their models among their age-mates on the playground and in school. When they are old enough to hear stories read or to see movies and television, they discover new heroes and heroines and pick new models. When they are able to read, their horizon broadens and their dreams of glory keep shifting with the levels of their understanding.

Changing interests result in part from disappointment and disillusion, for while parents may praise a good try at acting like a space man or a movie star, each child discovers that some of his friends are able to do even better than he. A child cannot win every athletic contest and every hand-to-hand fight. The best that parents can do is to encourage a child in whatever he tries while helping him to accept the failures for what they are—a part of learning about his limitations. At the same time they can suggest other worthwhile activities that are within the range of his abilities and interests. Although the childish values and strivings are eventually outgrown, many children need help in discovering what is most worthwhile to them.

Some children set their goals in terms of what they can do easily and well, without any sense of rivalry and also without much concern about the value of their efforts. However excellent their achievements may turn out to be, such individuals are in effect withdrawing themselves from any kind of competition. A scholarly monk or a fine painter or a creative scientist can justify himself by the purity of his motives, for he strives for excellence for its own sake.

Parents sometimes complain that a boy or girl lacks ambition. This usually means that the child has failed to become sufficiently interested in any one aspect of life to want to do something about it. He may have experienced too many frustrations in efforts already made, or the competition may have been too great. He may have dreams that seem utterly unattainable, that could not be understood or appreciated. In some cases, bodily conditions may account for indifference or lack of purpose.

A child who is considered "too ambitious" may be one whose energies have not found sufficient outlets and is eager to be noticed.

Parents have their own ambitions and ideas and often would like to fulfill themselves in the achievements of their children, especially if they have themselves been frustrated. They can be most helpful, however, if they treat each child as a distinct person and try to find the best use for his own combination of talents and shortcomings. *See also* AGGRESSIVENESS.

AMBIVALENCE, the coexistence within a person of opposite or conflicting feelings, such as love and hate. It refers to impulses, conscious or unconscious, that contradict each other and may be symptomatic of schizophrenia. *See also* SCHIZOPHRENIA.

AMEBIASIS, an infection caused by an organism called *endamoeba histolytica. Amebic dysentery* usually develops and occasionally the condition spreads to the liver, in which case *amebic hepatitis* follows.

The chief symptom of amebic dysentery is *diarrhea,* which becomes increasingly acute for three or four days and is accompanied by weakness, nausea, vomiting, and cramps, felt mostly on the right side of the body. Fever occurs infrequently. The infecting organism invades the body as tiny cysts which are able to resist both freezing and chlorine in the concentration usually used for purifying water. The amebae travel to the colon and infect the mucous surface of the wall, eventually creating abscesses of varying severity. The organisms may live in the intestines for months without producing serious consequences, and the infection may become widespread before any evident symptoms appear. Once the attacks of dysentery begin, they may recur at intervals and in the intervening periods the infected person will have various intestinal disturbances. If untreated the disease may cause anemia and emaciation. Treatment with *emetine, iodine, terramycin, arsenical compounds,* or new drugs like *milibis* usually produces satisfactory results. Amebic dysentery resembles *bacillary dysentery* and other acute intestinal infections. The diagnosis must be made on the basis of a microscopic examination of the infected person's excretions.

Amebic hepatitis, or abscess of the liver, involves pain, irregular fever, and tenderness of the liver. It occurs when amebae present in an intestinal infection migrate to the liver, though two-thirds of those with amebic hepatitis do not have dysentery. Abscesses are treated by surgical methods. *See also* LIVER, COMMON DISEASES OF; AMEBIC DYSENTERY; BACILLARY DYSENTERY; DIARRHEA. *See* MEDIGRAPH page 167.

► Transmissible Diseases, *Amebiasis and Dysentery,* 2316.

AMEBIC DYSENTERY, inflammation of the colon, caused by invasion of a single-celled parasite, *endamoeba histolytica.* It has been estimated that from 1.5 to 10 per cent of the population of the United States is infested with this parasite, which enters the body in contaminated food and drink. Amebic dysentery is more prevalent in economically poor areas and in hot climates.

Symptoms of amebic dysentery may be mild, with only fatigue and depression, or may include constipation, nausea, slight appetite, gas, and abdominal cramps. When the organisms spread throughout the wall of the bowel, there is severe diarrhea with excretion of blood, pronounced weakness, prostration, vomiting and pain on the right side of the abdomen. Usually fever is not present or only slight.

Recovery is slow and the condition may become chronic, with anemia and occasional occurrences of more severe diarrhea. When the dysentery is not cured, the organisms enter the liver and lungs and form abscesses.

Amebic dysentery is often difficult to control and it may be necessary to repeat the treatment. One method of management is to give the patient a dose of castor oil, followed by iodine-containing compounds for eight or ten days, with a diet of milk and milk products until the acute phase has passed. *Aureomycin* and *terramycin* have also proved effective. If the liver and lungs have been invaded, special drugs are given.

The organisms causing amebic dysentery are hard to destroy, and can be carried on fruit, vegetables, flies, cockroaches, and water. Careful personal and public cleanliness is the best means of avoiding the disease. *See also* BACILLARY DYSENTERY; DIARRHEA; AMEBIASIS. *See* MEDIGRAPH page 167.

AMENORRHEA, absence of menstruation, either normal cessation or suppression. *See also* MENSTRUATION.

AMENTIA, subnormal mental development. It is mental deficiency, such as idiocy, which begins in infancy, adolescence, or is congenital. Amentia is contrasted with dementia. *See also* DEMENTIA; FEEBLEMINDEDNESS.

the disease and its causes Amebiasis or amebic dysentery is caused by amebae—microscopic one-celled animals. This disease affects about 10% of the population of the United States and is found throughout the world, particularly in warmer climates. Primarily, the bowels are involved, but the disease may affect other organ systems, particularly the liver and the lungs.

Infected flies, water, and food are among the transmitting agents. Infected food handlers are particularly responsible. The disease is common in areas where human waste is used for fertilizer.

Once the ameba has been eaten, or otherwise taken internally, it lodges in the lower end of the small intestine. Here it develops, multiplies, and ultimately becomes capable of penetrating the bowel wall and spreading to other parts of the body. Some of these amebae may be excreted with the stool. In the cyst form the disease is contagious.

The incubation period varies from a few days, which is the usual time, to from nine to eighty days.

symptoms There is great variation in the severity of the symptoms. Many individuals who are carriers never know it and never have any symptoms. In the acute form, the onset is sudden. There is severe abdominal pain, nausea, vomiting, and liquid stools with blood and mucus excreted up to 15-20 times a day. Marked rectal pain accompanies the bowel movements. If there is any fever it is mild, but the patient feels weaker and weaker.

In most cases, the attack leaves the patient with chronic amebic dysentery with characteristic bouts of diarrhea from time to time, gas, loss of appetite and weight, weakness, usually some anemia and periods of low-grade fever. Without treatment the condition may last for years and the patient can become a chronic invalid.

complications Liver involvement occurs in about 5% of all cases of amebiasis, with abscess of the liver the most serious and common complication. When the abscess ruptures there is peritonitis and the outlook becomes much more serious.

Another complication is involvement of the right lung and pleural cavity, usually by direct extension from amebic liver disease. The patient develops lung abscess and empyema (which is an accumulation of pus in the pleural sac).

The pericardium, which is the sac containing the heart, can be affected. Painful, destructive skin lesions can also occur.

prevention (or lessening of impact) The doctor can detect amebic infection by stool examination, or proctoscopic study. Specific drugs are available to eradicate amebae from the large bowel and treat any liver involvement.

In areas where amebic infection exists, care must be given to the protection of the water supply and to proper sewage disposal. People in these areas should also avoid eating fresh, uncleaned vegetables, and should protect food from flies.

Amebiasis and Amebic Dysentery

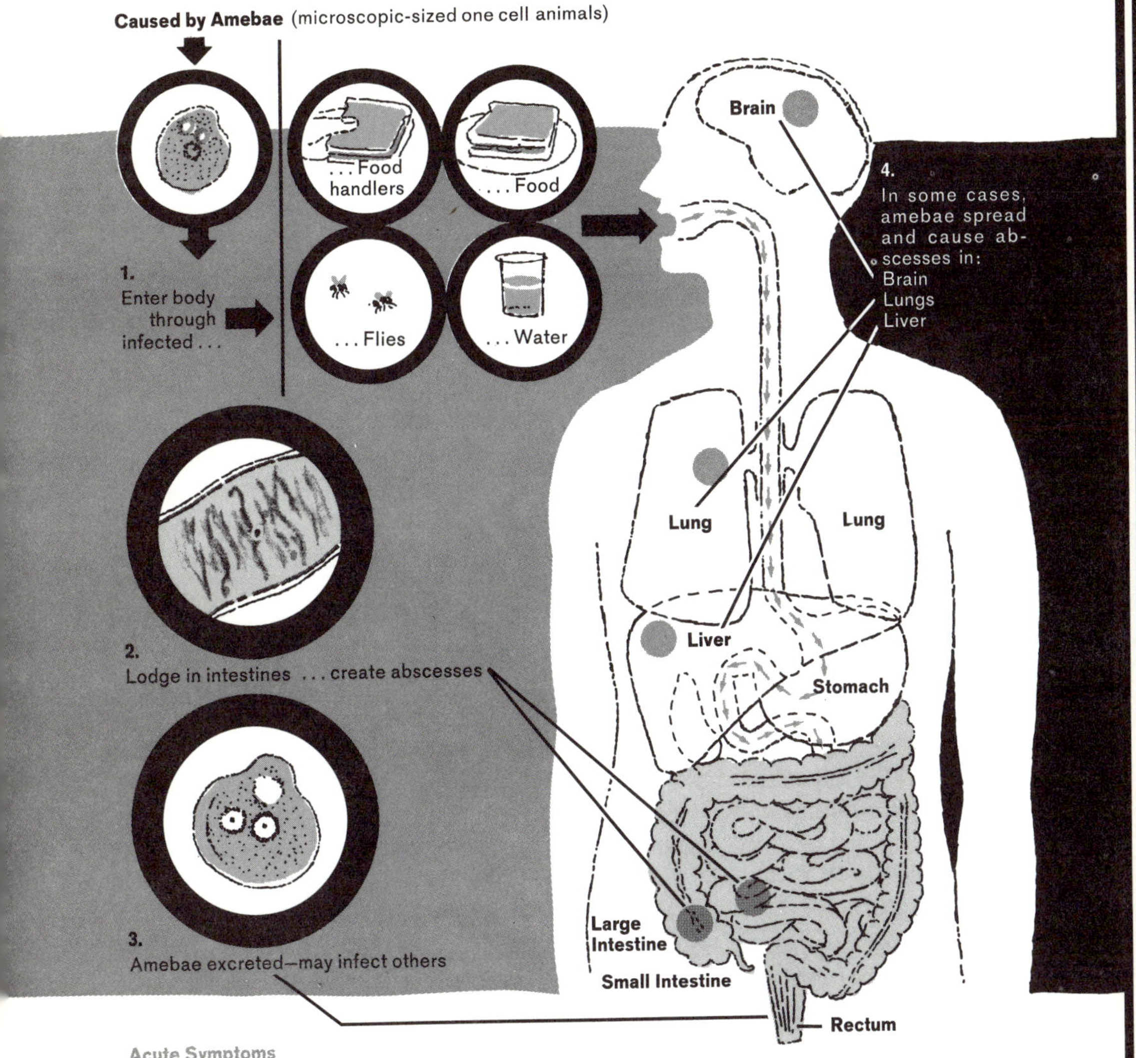

Enter body through infected . . .

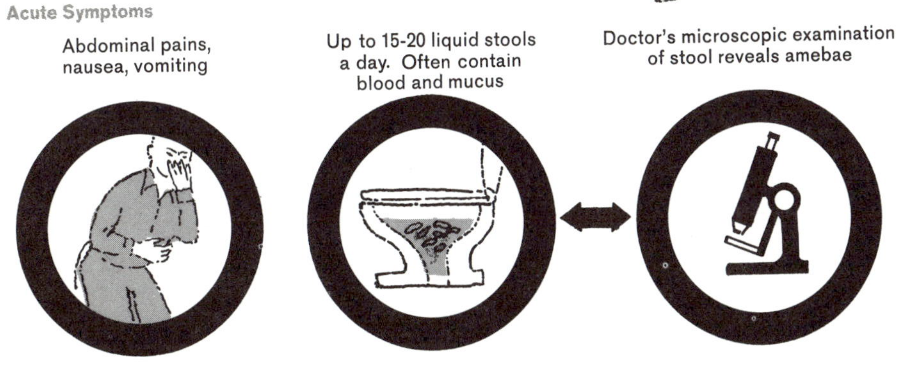

Lodge in intestines . . . create abscesses

Amebae excreted—may infect others

In some cases, amebae spread and cause abscesses in:

Acute Symptoms
Abdominal pains, nausea, vomiting
Up to 15-20 liquid stools a day. Often contain blood and mucus
Doctor's microscopic examination of stool reveals amebae

AMERICAN HEART ASSOCIATION. The evolution of our knowledge of heart disease, how to diagnose it, how to treat it, how to predict the future, has advanced tremendously in recent years. The fears that formerly prevailed have been dissipated. The campaign of public education conducted by the American Heart Association, public participation by the donating of funds, the establishment of a National Heart Institute in which government funds are used directly for heart research and for giving grants to workers in various universities, have all contributed to our advancement. All this has combined in accelerating the pace of research, in giving physicians sufficient tools for work with patients and in giving patients the opportunity for years free from pain and distress.

AMINO ACIDS, organic compounds often called the building blocks of protein. They are absorbed into the blood from the digestive tract and distributed throughout the body to the tissues, which use them to build new proteins. Protein is essential to the living cells. The body uses amino acids to replace the parts of the body proteins which are constantly being destroyed or lost.

Amino acids are supplied primarily by meat, fish, poultry, cheese, milk, and eggs. They contain carbon, hydrogen, oxygen, and nitrogen, and sometimes sulphur. Their composition, as they are found in the food proteins, is the same as that of the amino acids present in the proteins of body tissues, although they have a different chemical construction. Some amino acids can be adequately manufactured from other materials in the body. Other amino acids cannot be manufactured within the body in sufficient quantity to supply the demands of growth and repair, and must be provided in the diet if the body is to survive. The supply of protein is considered adequate when the nitrogen balance of the body is maintained. The amino acids that are indispensable for the maintenance of nitrogen balance are *arginine, histidine, lysine, leucine, isoleucine, methionine, phenylalanine, trytophane, threonine,* and *valine.*

Preparations of different amino acids are available commercially. These preparations contain the amino acids in the same proportions as are produced by the breakdown of proteins, and they are used to supplement the dietary nitrogen in readily assimilable form. They are essential in the treatment of severe protein deficiency, in conditions in which food is not assimilated normally, and after surgical operations which involve the alimentary tract. *See also* NUTRITION; PROTEIN; VITAMINS.

AMINOPHYLLINE, or *theophylline ethylenediamine,* a yellowish white powder with a bitter taste generally used in conditions affecting the heart in pulmonary congestion and in the treatment of asthma.

This drug may be given by slow injection into the veins and occasionally is prescribed as a rectal suppository. *See also* ANGINA PECTORIS; ASTHMA.

AMINOPTERIN, a synthetic drug, one of the so-called *folic acid antagonists* developed in the search for effective treatment in acute leukemia. The folic acid antagonists counteract the abnormal increase in white cells which characterizes leukemia, and aminopterin has been found to be the most effective of them. Growing experience with the use of this drug, later alternated with *ACTH* or *cortisone,* has resulted in lengthening the periods of improvements which now last as long as three years. Aminopterin is also used to treat some other forms of cancer. *See also* LEUKEMIA; WHITE BLOOD CELLS, DISEASES OF.

AMMONIA, a highly irritating poisonous gas, easily soluble in water; forms *ammonium hydroxide,* widely employed in medicine and in the household. Ammonia is a strong and rapidly acting stimulant used in smelling salts for relief in cases of fainting or exhaustion. The solution and vapors are extremely irritating to the mucous membranes, and concentrated solutions will burn the tissues, as do all corrosive poisons. The antidote for ammonia poisoning is olive oil taken by mouth with large quantities of water, or weak vinegar or lemon juice in water. *See also* POISONING.

AMNESIA, loss of memory, especially inability to recognize ideas represented by words.

The symptoms of amnesia are varied and of different types. *Anterograde amnesia* is loss of memory directly following severe shock or trauma. *Auditory amnesia* is an inability to recognize the spoken word. In *retrograde amnesia,* memory of all previous events is obliterated, and sometimes those incidents occurring after an accident are also effaced (*post-traumatic amnesia*). The latter is of variable duration and is a yardstick of the severity of the shock or injury.

Amnesia may be *partial*—as, for instance, losing one's memory for sounds, names, or colors—or it may be *general* with a loss of the greater part of memory. It frequently involves a sudden emotional conflict, and memory will begin to return when the conflict is resolved. Doctors often find it difficult to decide in these cases whether or not the inability to remember is actual or simulated. If someone simply refuses to remember, the diagnosis is difficult. Cases are on record of persons who have had as many as five periods of complete loss of memory with subsequent recovery.

Occasionally one reads of a person who cannot recall his name or address. Psychiatrists believe that such persons suffer from amnesia because of their inability to cope with situations which apparently were so painful that the only solution was to deny their identity.

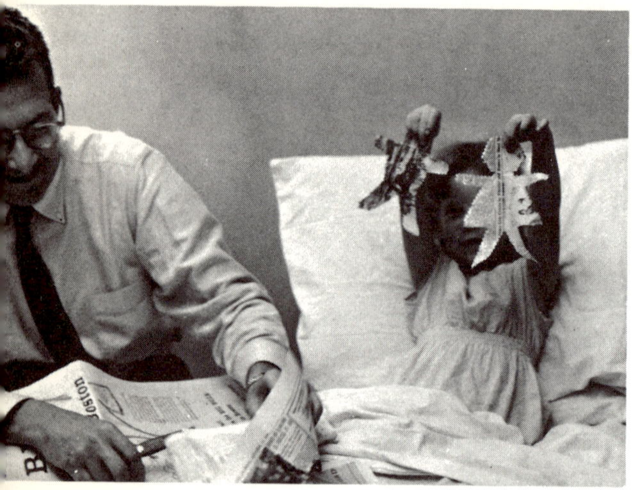

Amusing the Sick Child – Constructive toys and materials, such as beads, slates, crayons and cutouts, will help the sick child to occupy his time. Although even the older child will need company, he must not expect his parents' constant attention.

Even in total amnesia certain habits are remembered, such as writing, walking, and reading.

AMNION, the inner fetal membrane of the sac or bag which encloses and protects the embryo. It contains the amniotic fluid which surrounds the fetus until the sac is ruptured at birth. *See also* CHILDBIRTH AND PRENATAL CARE; UTERUS.

AMOG. This is a term derived from the Malay language similar to the English "amuck." The term "running amuck" refers to a condition of hysterical excitement which follows an infectious disease such as malaria or brooding on personal relationships. There is a condition called *latah* which begins with a shriek, after which the victim may imitate everything that is said and done.

AMPHETAMINE. *See* BENZEDRINE.

AMPUTATION, the removal of a limb or an organ of the body, in whole or in part. *See also* ARTIFICIAL LIMBS.

AMUSING THE SICK CHILD. While a child is really sick and without energy, he is content to sleep or lie quietly in his bed with a favorite toy to comfort him. When he starts to get better, however, some planning is necessary to furnish amusements that will keep him quietly occupied until his full energy has returned. More planning is needed, of course, for younger children than for those over 10 or so. Older boys and girls have their hobby materials or collections or may ask that the phonograph be played or try to use the time to catch up on schoolwork. Some are content for long periods with a bedside radio or television and favorite books or comics.

For younger patients there is a wide variety of play materials—including ordinary household articles—that can provide fun in bed.

A gay mobile dancing in front of a window is fun for anyone to watch. Some children are content for an interval with dolls to dress and undress; miniature autos, trains, or trucks to be maneuvered amid the bedclothes; jigsaw puzzles; scrapbooks and coloring books; old magazines and a pair of unpointed scissors; models of farm animals, airplanes, boats to put together.

Small children find entertainment in stringing big wooden beads or scribbling on a small hand slate with a piece of chalk.

It is necessary to provide adequate support for the child's back when he sits up in bed and sufficient lighting to prevent eyestrain. A large lightweight tray on legs or a sturdy low cardboard box with a knee-hole opening makes a convenient play surface. A shoe bag attached to the bedside serves as storage space for small play materials. A shopping bag looped over the bedpost makes a handy catch-all for debris. A sheet or a blanket cover protects blankets.

In spite of the extra attention that a sick child gets, he is likely to become lonely now and then. Even the older boy or girl naturally wants company some of the time—for a game of cards or checkers, or just a chat. Fixing up a special bed for a youngster near the area where his mother spends most of her time is often a happy answer to the situation. If he must remain in his own room, however, it's easier to keep him quietly in bed when his mother finds short periods for reading to him, telling him stories, or playing games; there is time for riddles and word games as she dusts and straightens his room, and maybe she can do the family mending companionably at his bedside. Father can give his own special twist to stories; he can be impressed by the child's magic tricks or bring in his own. The young patient must be helped to understand that he cannot expect one of his parents to amuse him all day long. Some of the time he must amuse himself. If the disease involved is not communicable, and if the doctor permits, a few of his friends may come to see him if they play quietly and don't stay so long that they tire him out.

Some boys and girls enjoy so much the extra attention and indulgence that come with being sick, they may have occasional "relapses." An objective attitude from parents that the illness was unfortunate—but something over and done with now—helps the youngsters to get over this. *See also* CONVALESCENCE.

AMYLASE, any enzyme which, through a reaction with water, breaks down starch into sugar.

AMYOTROPHIC DISEASES, those disorders that cause degeneration of muscle. Degeneration and hardening of portions of the spinal cord which is promptly reflected in the muscles of the body is called *amyotrophic lateral sclerosis.*

The spinal cord is only eighteen inches long in a full-grown man and weighs less than one ounce. It is, therefore, much shorter than the spinal or vertebral column in which it lies. The tissue of the spinal cord is divided into parts which are anterior, meaning the front; lateral, meaning on the side; and posterior, meaning the back.

Obviously whenever there is a change of any kind in these tissues, the effects on the human body are far-reaching and serious. When something happens to the nervous tissues, the muscles which are controlled by this nervous tissue are likewise affected. The cause of amyotrophic lateral sclerosis is unknown. It is apparently not due to any well-established condition affecting the blood, and certainly there has been shown to be no infectious cause. It has been suggested that there are conditions within the body at birth which ultimately reveal themselves in this disease. The condition is seen mostly in mature age, usually between forty-five and sixty years of age, and affects men more often than it does women.

The chief symptoms are a progressive twitching of the muscles with increasing weakness and wasting away. The symptoms of the condition seem to be occasionally foreshadowed by vague feelings of exhaustion, occasional cramps, numbness, and a burning sensation. Usually, however, the patient comes to the doctor because he has noticed a gradual wasting of the muscles of one or both hands with twitching. From this point on progressive weakness and wasting are the most important symptoms.

The condition is seldom painful, although in some instances there may be severe pains. Unfortunately the condition does not tend to improve; the progressive wasting of the muscles and, associated therewith, inability of motion or action continue. Treatment helps to maintain the tone of the muscles and to alleviate worry. *See also* LATERAL SCLEROSIS.

► Diseases of the Nervous System, *Amyotrophic Lateral Sclerosis,* 1644.

ANALGESIA, insensibility to pain. It may be produced by drugs known as *analgesics* or by *nerve block.* Analgesic drugs relieve pain without producing loss of consciousness. Among the milder analgesics are *acetylsalicylic acid,* commonly known as *aspirin,* and *acetophenetidin,* or *phenacetin,* both of which may be obtained without a prescription. However, recent investigations indicate that these drugs should be used with caution, and should be kept inaccessible to children.

Among the stronger analgesics, used for the relief of severe pain, are *morphine, opium,* and *codeine,* all habit-forming drugs, which should be used only under the supervision of a physician. *See also* ANESTHESIA; MEDICINE CHEST, *Pain Relievers.*

ANAPHIA, a defective or absent sense of touch, or an abnormal sensitivity to touch.

ANAPHYLAXIS, the opposite of *immunity.* It denotes abnormal sensitivity and susceptibility to infection. *See also* IMMUNITY.

ANATOMY. The science of the structure of the body and the relation of its parts. Physicians use anatomical terms in describing the body and the relation of one part to another. Some of the more familiar anatomical terms are: anterior, toward the front side of the body; posterior, toward the back side of the body; medial, nearer the middle of the body; lateral, farther from the midline; internal, inside; external, outside; proximal, closer to the body; distal, away from the body; superior, above; inferior, below; cranial, toward the head; caudal, toward the lower end of the body.

ANCYLOSTOMA DUODENALE, a hookworm which thrives chiefly in man, though lower animals can play host to it. It is also an infestation by hookworms. *See also* WORMS.

ANDROGEN, a male hormone that produces and controls the secondary male sex characteristics, such as the beard, muscles, and deep voice. The male sex hormone *testosterone* is the primary androgen. The secretions produced by the testes include the androgens. *See also* HORMONES.

ANDROGYNY, or *pseudohermaphroditism,* is the state of having congenitally malformed external genitalia resembling those of one sex while the gonads are those of the opposite sex. *See also* HERMAPHRODITISM.

ANEMIA. In a healthy body, a balance is maintained between productive and destructive blood processes. Anemia, which occurs when the concentration of *hemoglobin* in the blood falls below a normal level, can result from any of a number of causes. Hemoglobin is the red coloring matter whose main function in the blood is to transport oxygen through the arteries to the body's cells. It is formed in the bone marrow and is normally found in the blood in a ratio of about 16 per cent. Anemia can be caused simply by loss of blood or it may result from a destruction of cells or from inadequate formation of cells. This may be due to some deficiency in nutrition as, for example, the lack of iron and protein or the special substance derived from the stomach or liver which is important for the formation of red blood cells. Apparently there are cases in which the thyroid gland is not sufficiently active to stimulate the mechanism involved.

Copper and cobalt are important in the formation of red blood cells. There are cases in which chemicals like benzene, arsenic, gold, and the sulfa drugs can damage the bone marrow so that it cannot produce cells adequately. There may also be damage by x-ray and radium or the growth of tumors in the bone marrow. To treat an anemic condition the doctor must first determine just what type of anemia it is and when this is established, correct the basic fault causing the anemia.

Anemias can follow a sudden blood loss from an injury or from internal hemorrhaging. In this case, the cells themselves are normal but reduced in number. Following a hemorrhage, the body compensates by adding fluids to the blood to re-

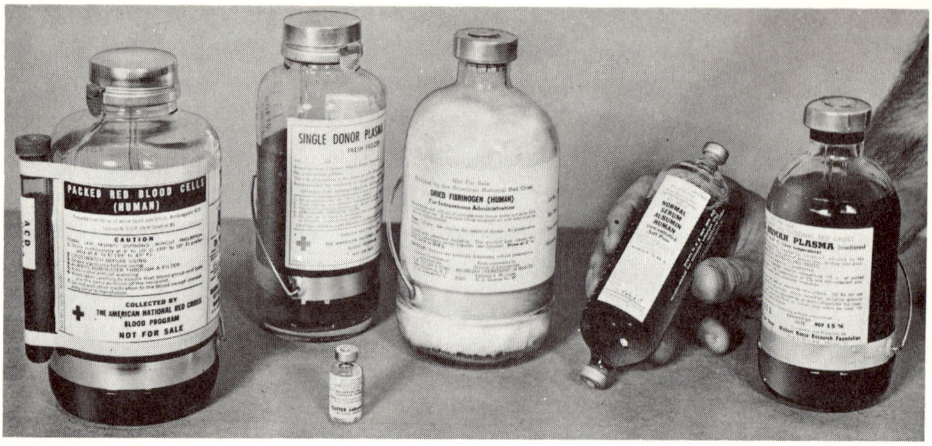

Anemia—With the use of modern separating machines and new chemical processes, whole blood can be broken down into many of its component parts. Some of these fractions are bottled and can be used to combat hemorrhage, anemia, shock, hepatitis, measles and poliomyelitis. Since only part of the blood may be needed in a given instance, this fractionation has resulted in the saving of much whole blood. However, in most anemias, especially anemia which occurs after bleeding, whole blood must still be used.

store it to its original volume. The blood is diluted by these fluids and the ratio of hemoglobin to total blood volume is lowered causing anemia. It often takes time for the body to manufacture sufficient red blood cells and other substances for the blood to become normal. Symptoms of blood loss anemia which result from the inability of the blood to carry enough oxygen include headache, general weakness, faintness, and dizziness. In more severe cases of blood loss, vomiting, intense thirst, a fast heart rate and weak shallow breathing as well as the other symptoms of shock are readily seen.

Treatment of this condition includes, of course, stopping the blood loss where such loss in evident—as in the case of wounds. Blood transfusions are sometimes given to prevent excessive dilution of the blood. In less serious hemorrhages, rest and proper diet, including iron and protein for building cells, will be sufficient to enable the body to restore the lost blood.

In a healthy body the life of a normal erythrocyte, or red blood cell is roughly 100 to 120 days. When it breaks down, hemoglobin is released. To make up for this loss, new red cells containing hemoglobin are constantly being manufactured to keep the hemoglobin content constant.

In anemia caused by abnormal breakdown or destruction of red blood cells, called *hemolytic anemia,* large hemoglobin is released at a much greater rate then it can be replaced. This is converted by the liver into other pigments excreted in the bile. When the manufacture of bile pigments is excessive, some appear in body tissue and give the skin and whites of the eyes a yellowish cast, the symptom commonly known as *jaundice.* In *hemolytic jaundice,* the cells are so fragile that they are broken down more rapidly than usual by the spleen. Without the spleen, the cells can function properly. The spleen may have to be removed in such cases to prevent the overly rapid cell disintegration.

Anemia is either congenital as in *sickle cell anemia* or may accompany various types of systemic diseases.

An excessive breakdown of red blood cells can also be caused by allergies, poisoning, malaria, severe burns and other conditions. The treatment in each case depends on the basic underlying cause.

Nutritional anemias, which are caused by deficiencies, are characterized by defective blood formation. Most common and least severe is the type in which the amount of iron, essential for hemoglobin manufacture, is inadequate. Eighty-five per cent of the iron necessary is released from the breakdown of old cells, but some iron must be supplied in the diet. Symptoms of *iron-deficiency anemia* commonly include pallor, weakness and fatigue, faintness and difficulty in breathing. It is easily diagnosed by laboratory tests and responds rapidly to proper diet and rest.

Anemia in a pregnant woman is caused by an attempt of her system to care more adequately for the growing baby. Since the blood of the woman must carry food, oxygen and waste products for two beings, de-

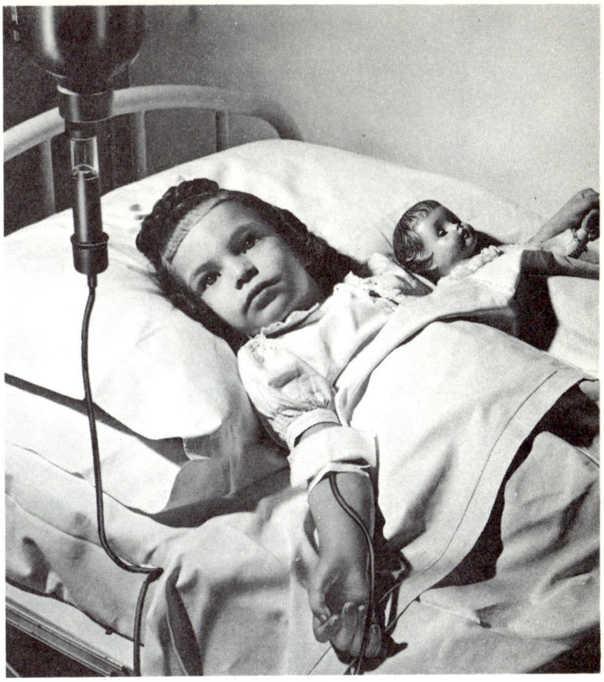

Anemia—Blood transfusions are given for many types of anemias. This little girl had received, up to the time the photograph was taken, 115 pints of blood.

mands on the circulatory system are increased, which can lead to a dilution of blood, with fewer red blood cells per cubic centimeter of blood. Inadequate diet or vomiting tend to increase the possibility of iron deficiency and the doctor may prescribe iron and protein supplements to the mother's diet. Normally, a baby is born with enough iron in his tissues to last several months but if the iron supply of the mother is low, the baby will have a low reserve and develop anemia unless diet supplements of iron are given. Milk is a poor source of iron. Copper, vitamin C and other vitamins are also thought to be involved in the body process of iron utilization.

Bone marrow deficiency disease is another anemia caused by defective blood formation from decreased bone marrow formation. The red

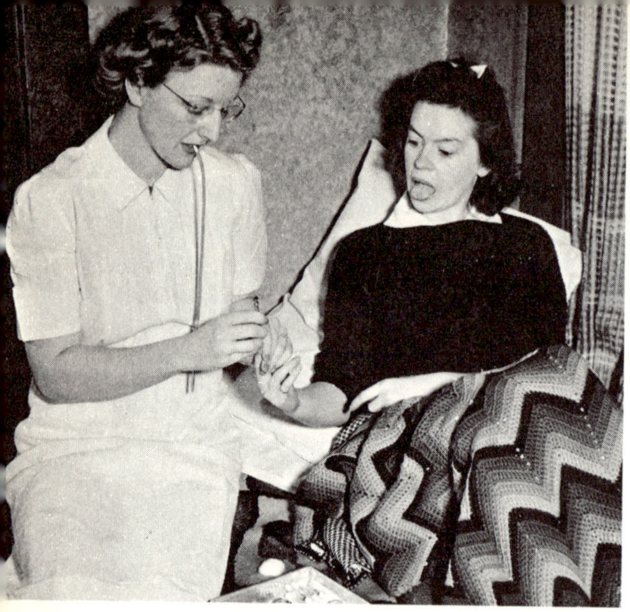

Anemia—With the few drops of blood she collects, the technician will determine the amount of hemoglobin present, the number of red and white corpuscles, and the kinds and proportions of different white corpuscles. These tests constitute a complete blood count. This procedure is the major method of diagnosing the presence of an anemia and its type. Many hospitals and physicians do complete blood counts on all patients as a matter of routine.

blood cell formation in bone marrow is highly complex and involves many functions of the body. In the marrow, the prospective red cells are larger than they will be when released and lack hemoglobin. Before the new cells are released into the blood stream, they shrink in size and gain hemoglobin. When something prevents normal development, or the cells are released prematurely, the result is oversized red cells. To mature properly, the cells must have a substance from the liver called the *growth* or *maturation factor.* This maturation factor is identical or closely related with vitamin B_{12}. To absorb vitamin B_{12}, the body uses a substance called the *intrinsic factor,* which is found in normal gastric juice. Some anemias are caused by absence of the intrinsic factor and others by a poor supply of the maturation factor.

Pernicious anemia is characterized by the disappearance of this intrinsic factor and, along with it, hydrochloric acid in the gastric juice. Therefore, vitamin B_{12} or the maturation factor cannot be absorbed and the red cells cannot mature properly. As pernicious anemia progresses, changes occur in the spinal column, with weakness and numbness of the limbs and eventually a complete loss of their control. As well as the other anemia symptoms of pallor, weakness and difficult breathing, there may be diarrhea, nausea, sore tongue and yellow pigmentation of skin.

No treatment is known to restore the intrinsic factor and hydrochloric acid to the gastric juice. However, in 1926, it was discovered that regular amounts of liver in the diet would control pernicious anemia. Today intramuscular injections of highly concentrated liver extract, sometimes in conjunction with vitamin B_{12} and folic acid, are given instead of liver. However, this is not a cure and must be continued through the lifetime of the person.

Many other conditions exist in which absorption of material from the intestine is impaired as a result of diarrhea, excess fat in the intestine or impairment of intestinal walls. Other anemias include *sprue, pellagra, infestation with fish tapeworm, liver disease, myxedema,* and rare ones whose causes are unknown. Most of these conditions respond favorably to liver injections alone or with vitamin B_{12}.

Probably the most serious of the anemias are those caused by destruction of bone marrow. Cells of all types rapidly disappear from the blood stream until only a small percentage of the normal amount is left. It may be attributable to overdose of radium, x-ray, or severe infection, but usually the cause of the destruction is not known. Sometimes an improvement or cure is effected by repeated blood transfusions.

All anemias are characterized by general weakness and fatigue, since the blood cannot supply body tissue with sufficient nourishment. If the anemia develops gradually, the number of red blood cells may fall from a normal of 6,000,000 to as low as 1,000,000 and the red coloring matter may be only 20 per cent. The hemoglobin, or red coloring matter of the blood, is measured by various techniques—the simplest being colored charts in which the color of a certain percentage of red coloring matter is said to be normal, the next 90 per cent, and so on down. By actual weight 15 grams (or ½ ounce of hemoglobin) for every 100 c.c. (or one-fifth of a pint) of blood is said to be normal. However, accurate measurement is exceedingly difficult, so that the usual color scales would probably register anything above 13½ grams as representing 100 per cent.

Treatment of anemic conditions is much more satisfactory and more rapid if it is begun before the disease has progressed far or done permanent damage and early discovery of the condition is of prime significance. Usually, diagnosis is made by a laboratory examination of the person's blood and often tests are also made of samples of digestive juice or bone marrow. After the cause has been removed, specific substances are available to bring quick relief in all but a few rare types of anemia. *See also* ANEMIA, PERNICIOUS; SPRUE; PELLAGRA; RED BLOOD CELLS, DISEASES OF; LIVER, COMMON DISEASES OF; MYXEDEMA. *See* MEDIGRAPHS pages 1489, 1967.

► The Blood and Its Diseases, *The Anemias,* 351; *Anemia Due to Lack of Iron,* 353; *The Anemia of Chronic Infection, Chronic Inflammation and Cancer,* 353; *Mediterranean Anemia,* 354; *Pernicious Anemia,* 354; *Aplastic Anemia,* 355.

ANEMIA, PERNICIOUS. Since 1822 it has been known that there is a condition in which the body fails to produce a sufficient number of red blood cells of a quality and character capable of supporting the health of the body. In that year a doctor described accurately a case of *pernicious anemia.* Then another doctor gave a well-nigh perfect description of the condition in 1849. The disease was considered to be incurable until 1926, when doctors found that a half pound of liver taken daily would control the condition.

Pernicious anemia rarely occurs before the age of thirty. Most of the cases develop in people past forty or fifty years of age.

Early it was recognized that some disturbance of the digestive system of the body is associated with pernicious anemia. For instance an *absence of hydrochloric acid* in the secretion of the stomach may appear years before the pernicious anemia and may continue even when treatment with liver has been carried on. It was found that the normal person has in the secretion of his stomach a certain substance called an *intrinsic factor*—that is, developed within the cells—which reacts with food to produce a substance that is necessary in maintaining the normal formation of blood. This substance is absorbed from the bowel and stored in the liver and other tissues. In pernicious anemia the substance is not present in the liver. The exact nature of this substance is not known but its absence will interfere with the formation of normal red blood cells.

The discovery of the method for saving the lives of people with pernicious anemia was most important because the death rate from that disease had been rising steadily. Today, as a result of the discovery of the treatment of pernicious anemia with liver extract, the death rate has dropped.

The person with pernicious anemia is pale and his skin develops a lemon-yellow color; the tongue gets sore at the edges. The condition comes on gradually with an increasing sense of fatigue and tiredness, weakness, shortness of breath, headaches, and disturbances of digestion. If the condition persists without control, the nervous system becomes affected. There is numbness and tingling of the arms and legs, eventually difficulty in walking and lack of control of the usual functions of the body. The liver and the spleen become enlarged. The red bone marrow becomes soft and of a deep red color. The onset of the condition has been described thus: "It makes its approach in so slow and insidious a manner that the patient can hardly fix a date to his earliest feeling of that languor which is shortly to become so extreme."

When the doctor examines the blood, he frequently finds that there is a greater reduction of the red cells than of the red coloring matter. Because of the insidious approach of the disease the red cells may drop to 2,500,000 before the person begins to realize that something is wrong.

Only since the invention of the microscope and the use of the laboratory for studying the composition and character of the blood has it been possible for physicians to make the kind of studies that are necessary in differentiating various blood diseases from each other. Now we know that there are many different forms of disturbances of the blood which may affect the fluid matter, the chemicals dissolved in the fluid, the red blood cells, the white blood cells of various types, the blood platelets or materials involved in causing the blood to clot.

In the most serious cases the doctor not only uses all these techniques to examine blood taken from a puncture of the ear or finger but he may actually take a sample of the bone marrow from the breastbone in order to determine whether or not any important changes have taken place in that blood-forming tissue. The doctor will not diagnose anemia from the blood alone because, as has already been shown, there are so many different kinds of anemia and because the treatment must be definitely related to the peculiar variety. Then again, the doctor is enabled to determine the nature of the anemia by studying the blood before and after the use of various forms of treatment. The giving of iron will bring about stimulation of the formation of red blood cells and of red coloring matter in the blood. The giving of liver extract will have a definite effect on the bone marrow when that substance is absent from the tissues of the body. Obviously the patient who is completely at rest while undergoing treatment is likely to recover much more rapidly than the one who tries to work or engage in other activities which may interfere with the forces of the body while treatment is going on. Then again the doctor who treats the patient with liver extract, iron, or both must determine exactly how much of each of these substances is necessary in an individual case. He must also determine the manner in which the material is to be given. We know from the results of experience that liver extract is sixty times as effective when given by injection into the body as when given by mouth. The injection may be made directly into the muscles and thus the action is prompt. It is known that a unit of liver extract injected daily into the muscles in a person whose red blood cells have fallen to 1,500,000 for each cubic millimeter of blood will cause an increase to about 2,500,000 red blood cells in each cubic millimeter of blood a month.

One of the most amazing sights in modern medicine is the rapidity with which patients improve once the diagnosis has been made and the treatment given by the doctor.

Associated with the administration of the liver extract there should be improvement in the diet by including liberal amounts of liver, green vegetables, and fruit. Occasionally doses of hydrochloric acid may be given to take the place of the hydrochloric acid that is absent from the stomach. If the condition is diagnosed early and proper treatment given soon, the majority of patients recover promptly. However, there is a tendency toward relapse, so that these patients should be seen regularly by the doctor over a considerable period of time.

Folic acid and the more recently discovered vitamin B_{12} have the power to stimulate formation of red blood cells far more powerfully than liver extract. With vitamin B_{12} the intrinsic factor of the stomach wall may be given. *See also* ANEMIA; RED BLOOD CELLS, DISEASES OF.

► The Blood and Its Diseases, *Pernicious Anemia,* 354.

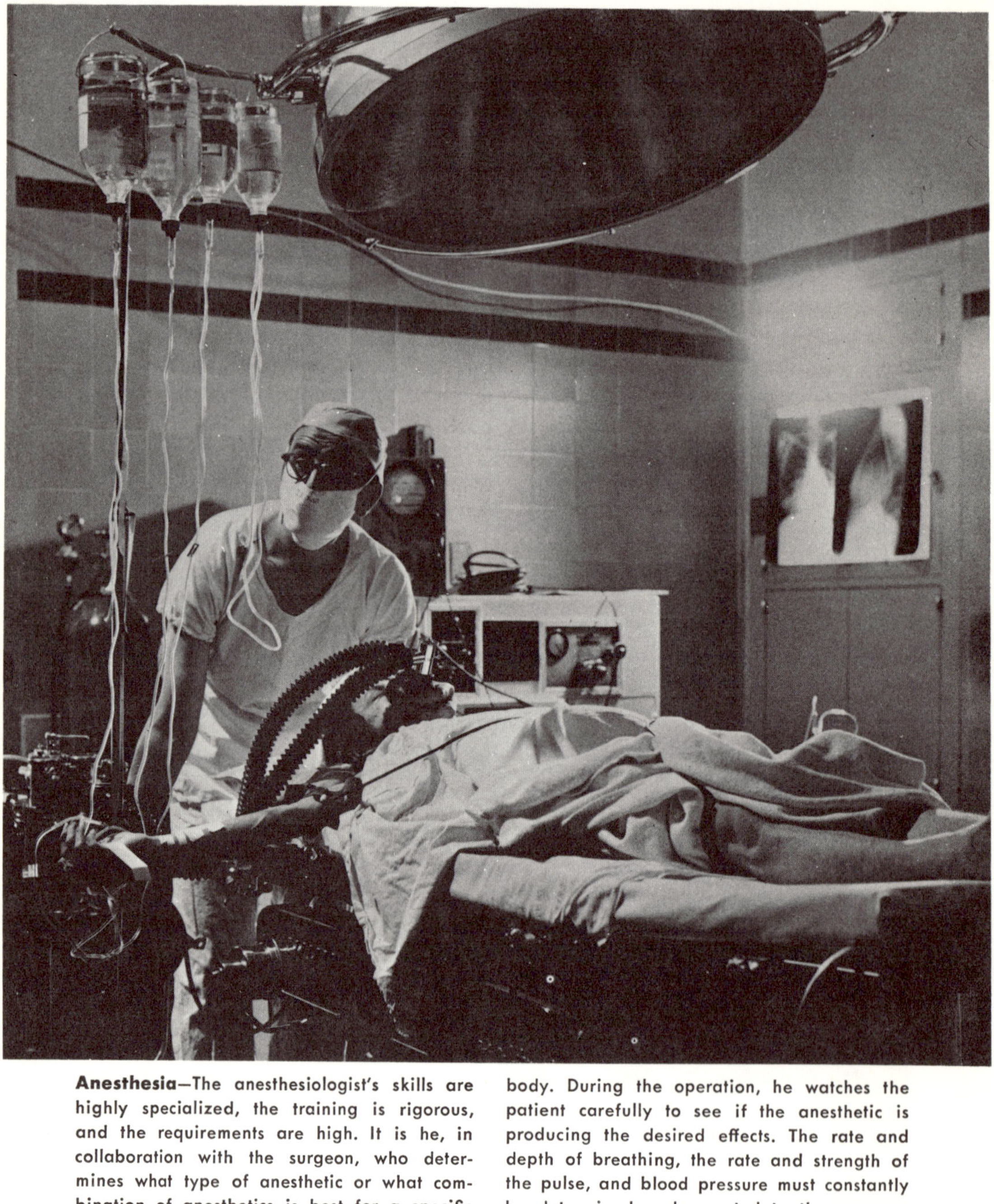

Anesthesia—The anesthesiologist's skills are highly specialized, the training is rigorous, and the requirements are high. It is he, in collaboration with the surgeon, who determines what type of anesthetic or what combination of anesthetics is best for a specific surgical procedure. In addition, his choice of anesthesia will depend on such factors as the patient's age and general condition of the body. During the operation, he watches the patient carefully to see if the anesthetic is producing the desired effects. The rate and depth of breathing, the rate and strength of the pulse, and blood pressure must constantly be determined and reported to the surgeon. The anesthesiologist must also administer blood transfusions and intravenous solutions when indicated by the patient's condition.

ANESTHESIA, a word first used in 1846 by Oliver Wendell Holmes, means the absence of pain sensation, with or without loss of consciousness. Three forms of insensibility to pain are recognized: (1) *general anesthesia,* loss of consciousness; (2) *regional* or *spinal anesthesia,* lack of pain in a limited area; and (3) *topical anesthesia,* lack of pain on a surface area by direct application of an anesthetic agent. The concept of anesthesia is ancient and *alcohol* and *opium* were used for many centuries to relieve pain.

Nitrous oxide, or *laughing gas,* was discovered by Joseph Priestley in 1769; and in 1799 another Englishman, Sir Humphry Davy, noted that nitrous oxide was able to produce unconsciousness. In 1844 an American dentist, Horace Wells, tested this property by having one of his own teeth painlessly removed while he was under the influence of nitrous oxide.

Ether, which was discovered in the sixteenth century, gained prominence in 1829 when Michael Faraday discovered that it produced unconsciousness. In 1842, a Georgia physician, Crawford W. Long, used ether successfully in an operation to remove a wen; and in 1846 a Boston dentist, William Thomas Green Morton, at Harvard, demonstrated again the anesthetic quality of ether during an operation to remove a tumor of the neck performed by Dr. John D. Warren.

Chloroform was discovered by Samuel Guthrie of New York in 1831. Chloroform is rarely used as an anesthetic in the United States today because it can depress the heart and cause severe damage to the liver and kidney.

Sigmund Freud first described the properties of *cocaine,* a drug with powerful pain-killing action, but did not go on to experiment with it. In 1884 Karl Koller of Vienna used cocaine in an operation on the eye, and it is now universally used as a local anesthetic by opthalmologists. Cocaine proved equally effective in producing local anesthesia on the mucous membranes of the nose, throat, and larynx. The discovery that cocaine was an anesthetic provoked many experiments in its use. Dr. William S. Halsted, an American physician, produced anesthesia of an entire area of the body by injecting cocaine into the nerve supplying the area. Dr. J. L. Corning introduced spinal anesthesia, which obtained insensibility of the entire lower part of the body. Further tests produced less toxic derivatives of cocaine and led to the development of *novocaine,* or *procaine,* which soon replaced all cocaine derivatives. At present, spinal anesthesia employing novocaine has become extensively used in operations for appendectomy, and on the lower abdomen and legs.

An outgrowth of spinal anesthesia was the development of *caudal anesthesia,* in which the anesthetic is injected into the sacral canal. In "painless childbirth," the anesthetic is injected in small amounts, a continuous "drip injection," into the region of the coccyx and acts on nerves leading to the womb.

Improvements in the methods of administering anesthetics have accompanied the discovery of safer drugs. One of the most significant steps has been the development of the "closed system" of administration. In the past, ether was given by dropping it into an open cone held over the patient's face. In the new system of administering ether, or supplementary gases, the gas is conducted through a series of closed tubes leading into a mask fitted tightly over the patient's face. This apparatus can absorb the carbon dioxide in the air exhaled by the patient, add oxygen when it is needed to the air inhaled, and add the anesthetic gases in the necessary concentrations. Anesthesia can thus be carried on for a much longer time and with much greater safety.

New and better anesthetics have continued to be developed. *Ethylene* and *cyclopropane* are in common use in many hospitals, although they have the one disadvantage, not yet completely overcome, of being highly explosive.

Another current method of administering an anesthetic is the intravenous or basal method in which the anesthetic drug is injected directly into the blood through the vein. The amount injected can be controlled by a stopcock on the needle and the anesthetic may be given in small amounts, thus keeping the patient free from pain for a long period of time. One of the first drugs used in this type of anesthesia was *evipal,* a barbiturate. Another more potent barbiturate now used is *pentothal sodium.*

The practice of anesthesia, which entails a knowledge of the proper administration of an anesthetic during an operation, the management of the patient's respiration, the ability to apply artificial respiration when necessary, and complete familiarity with the problems of gas therapy, has become a special field of medicine. Specialists who deal solely with this field are known as anesthetists or anesthesiologists.

► Drugs and Their Uses, *Anesthetics,* 900.

ANEURYSM, dilation of an artery or vein caused when a weak spot occurs in the wall. The layers of elastic tissue that form the wall enable the vessels to dilate and contract. When they are stretched at any point, because of innate weakness, the enfeebled section pouches out and causes distention, just as in the weakened wall of a rubber tire.

This thinning out, which destroys a section of the elastic tissue, may be the result of an infection such as pneumonia, of a streptococcal or staphylococcal infection. Often physical injury to an arterial wall leaves it so weakened that an aneurysm may eventually occur. If the blood-filled sac ruptures, a serious, often fatal hemorrrhage may ensue.

Aneurysms are of various types. When one of the layers of tissue of the wall of the blood vessel also becomes the wall of the sac, a *true aneurysm* results. *False aneurysms* occur when the layers of the artery are all ruptured, leaving the surrounding tissues to retain the blood. Also the blood may force its way between layers of the arterial wall and separate them.

All arteries are subject to aneurysms, and a most commonly affected artery is the *aorta,* the large artery leading from the heart. The disorder may develop in a blood vessel as the result of an injury, and even though such aneurysms are smaller they are no less dangerous, and may prove fatal when they occur in the heart, brain, or other vital organ.

Should the aneurysm become greatly enlarged, pressure is exerted and crowds the area in which it occurs, such as the abdominal or chest cavity. Aneurysms may be painful, or produce difficulty in breathing, *dyspnea,* by pressing against the air passages, or cause swelling.

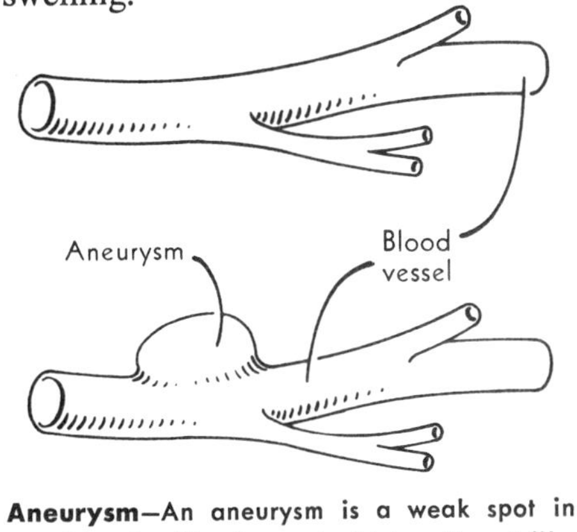

Aneurysm—An aneurysm is a weak spot in the side of a blood vessel which puffs out like a balloon.

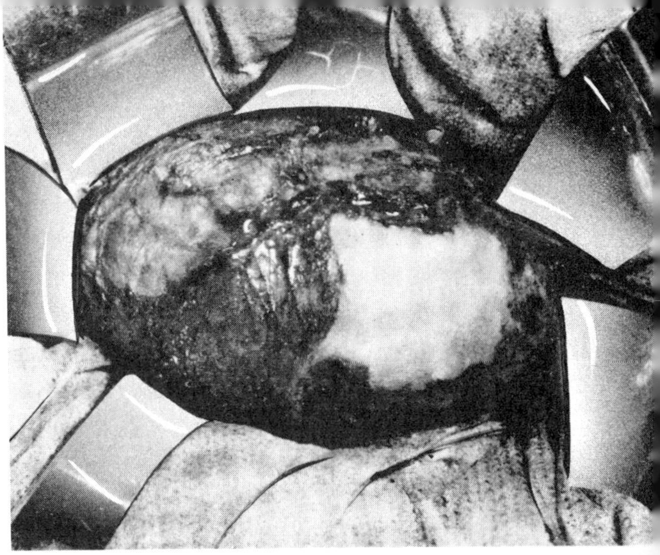

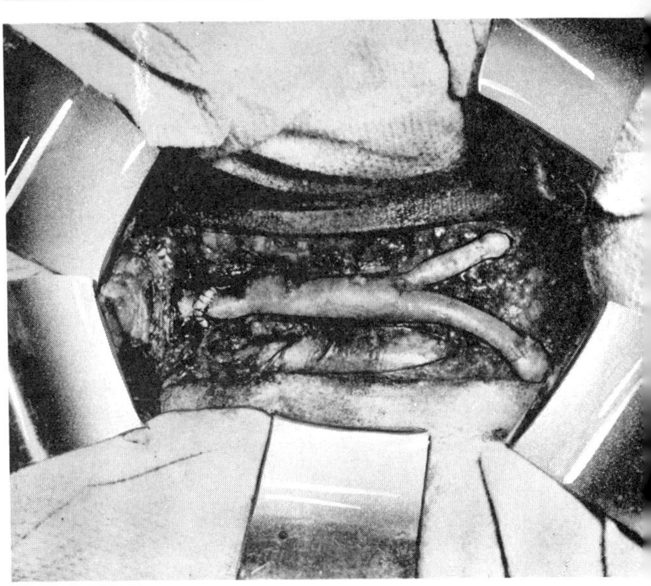

Aneurysm—An aneurysm may form in any artery of the body. A common site is in the aorta. A very large aneurysm of the aorta in the abdomen is shown *(top)* before surgery. The aneurysm has been removed and the damaged area of the aorta repaired *(bottom)*. In the past, treatment for an aneurysm was not very satisfactory and death often resulted. Today, gratifying results are being achieved with new and improved techniques for removing aneurysms and repairing vessels.

New techniques of surgery have been developed to repair the damaged artery walls. Smaller blood vessels are tied off and other arteries take over their function. It is also possible to coagulate the blood in

the disease and its causes An aneurysm is a sac formed by the enlargement of the wall of a blood vessel. This is caused by the destruction of elastic tissue in the artery or vein involved during the course of diseases such as arteriosclerosis, hypertension, and syphilis. The most important aneurysms are those which affect the important aortic artery, the main trunk of the entire arterial system.

Aneurysms vary in degree from slight widening of the blood vessel to an enlargement great enough to involve the ribs, esophagus, and lungs. They may be single or multiple, and of varying shapes. Frequently they are filled with large thrombi, or blood clots.

Older people subject to the diseases noted above are affected, as a rule, with a slightly higher frequency of aneurysms occurring in men than in women.

symptoms Symptoms depend upon the size and location of the aneurysm, although many aneurysms are present without any symptoms at all. However, when there is compression, or displacement, or interference with circulation to adjacent body structures, the aneurysm causes chronic disabilities. Those on the front part of the aorta may cause erosion of the ribs and even some bulging of the front chest wall. Chronic cough, frequent pneumonias, blood spitting, and a picture that resembles lung cancer may reveal the presence of an aneurysm in the arch of the aorta that is compressing the bronchial tubes. Further symptoms may be hoarseness, difficulty in swallowing, swelling of the neck, and perhaps swelling of an upper extremity.

Still other aneurysms can cause pain in the spine and nerves, high blood pressure, or kidney failure—as shown in the Medi-Graph.

complications The most serious complication occurs when the sac bursts. The result is hemorrhage and death. Depending upon the size and site of the aneurysm, other complications can develop. These include pulmonary infection, congestive heart failure, kidney failure, and circulatory problems of the extremities.

prevention (or lessening of impact) Aneurysms resulting from syphilis can be prevented by therapy with anti-syphilitic drugs during the early stages of this illness. Once a syphilitic aneurysm has formed, the doctor still prescribes treatment with these anti-syphilitic drugs—but how effective they will be depends upon how far along the disease has progressed. The drugs may relieve some of the symptoms and slow down further enlargement, but they will not cure the deformity already there.

There is no known way of preventing aneurysms that result from arteriosclerosis. The only treatment at present is surgery in which the diseased part of the blood vessel is replaced. Associated symptoms and complications are treated as they become evident.

Aneurysms

Bulging of blood vessel wall because of weak spot or loss of elasticity that develops. Bursting of sac can cause death

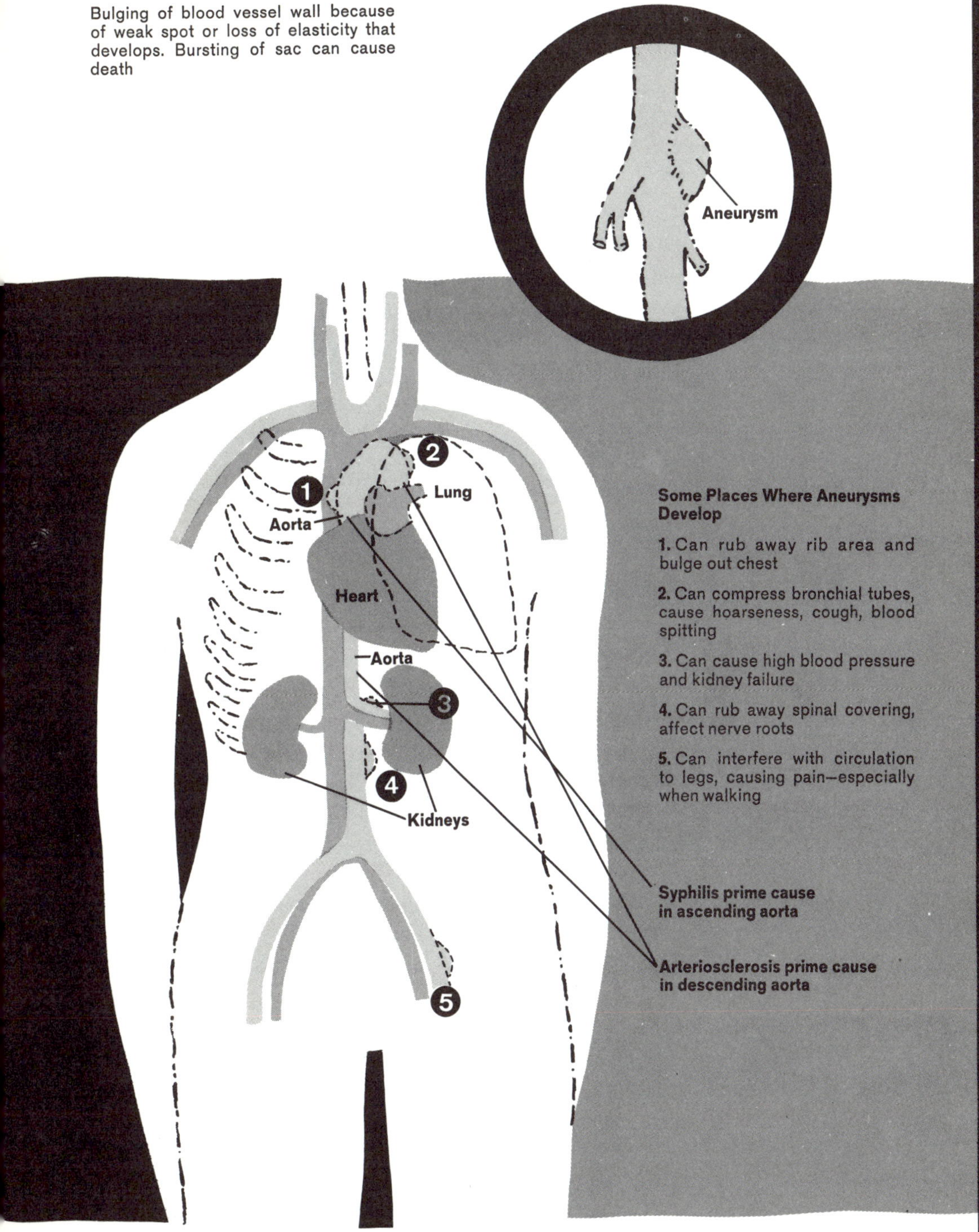

Some Places Where Aneurysms Develop

1. Can rub away rib area and bulge out chest

2. Can compress bronchial tubes, cause hoarseness, cough, blood spitting

3. Can cause high blood pressure and kidney failure

4. Can rub away spinal covering, affect nerve roots

5. Can interfere with circulation to legs, causing pain—especially when walking the sac and form a clot and thus strengthen the walls. Plastic materials are used around the aneurysm to prevent its growth, giving the weakened arterial wall opportunity to strengthen. *See also* CIRCULATORY SYSTEM; BACTERIAL ENDOCARDITIS. *See* MEDIGRAPHS pages 185, 287.

ANGER. A child has the right to be angry as much as he has the "right" to love. How his natural display of anger is treated during the years of childhood determines how he will use it in his adult life. It can be turned into channels like bullying, malice, prejudice, or petty criticism, or it can mature into a direct and strong attitude and method of protecting personal rights and opposing injustice.

Trying to "civilize" young children by teaching them to repress or hide their anger is a mistake. If anger cannot come out directly, it will find an outlet by turning on people or objects, or even by turning on oneself. In this case it may come out in physical illness, a result of tension set up by turning inward the anger that has not been permitted open expression. Children need to feel that when they show anger it is not in itself "bad"; that it is sometimes as natural for them to be angry as to smile.

Of course, as a child grows older, things that arouse his anger will change. The infant howls when his bottle is delayed too long; the toddler, having had some experience with delays, can wait a while for his meal. On the other hand, he may scream and stamp when he has to leave the playground, because he hasn't yet learned that if dinner is not to be delayed *he* has to be on time too. Some two years later he will have found out that everyone goes home to eat, that other children don't stay in the playground all night but do come back another day. By the time he is an adolescent, his anger can be aroused not only on behalf of himself or other individuals, but on behalf of causes, ideals, and groups of people all over the world.

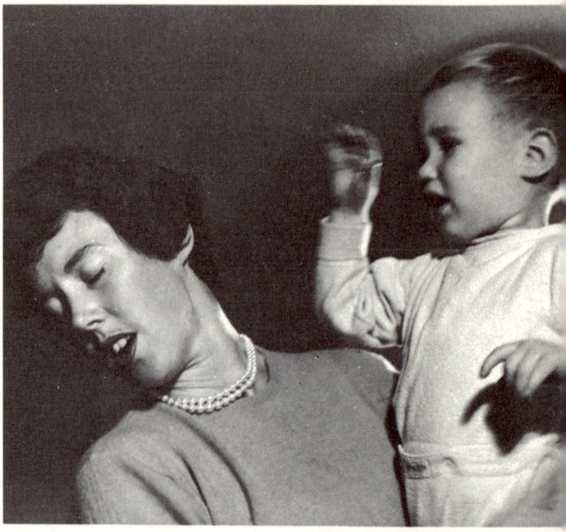

Anger — A child must learn, step by step, from parents and the world outside, to control anger. But he must feel free to express his feelings of anger. Repressed anger can emerge as bullying or malice, or may be turned inward on the child himself.

Gradually, step by step, a child learns to control and direct his anger. A toddler often strikes at another child or at an adult. Hitting out is his direct (and sometimes only) way of saying, "I'm mad!"

Soon he learns from other children that if he strikes he must expect to be struck back. He learns from grownups that while his anger in itself may be acceptable, his way of expressing it is not. "I won't let you hit me," states his father, holding the small hand firmly. A child can, perhaps, vent his feelings on a hammer toy, or pound away at a clay figure; but he will be stopped from pounding his little sister.

Learning to speak is a tremendous advance, for it is obviously more acceptable to express anger in words than by hitting and kicking and howling. The youngster can blow off steam and at the same time put into words for himself what is making him angry. Some adults tend to go too far by trying to put the child's thought into words for him. To say, "Yes, I know you hate me—it's all right," can be a dangerous practice. For one thing, the person who thus puts a child's feelings into words for him may be giving a completely inaccurate interpretation. The child may not hate the adult at all. For another, even if the child does have the feeling of hating the adult at the moment, this is quite different from having the person *tell* him he hates, which can be very frightening; and it's a quite different thing from the child himself spontaneously blurting out, "I hate you!" If the child's anger has always been accepted and treated honestly and naturally, he will feel free to put it into words himself. When he first does so he may need the help of being told, "I guess you do feel that way now." This has a double implication: that the child has a right to his feelings, and that his parents know he doesn't always feel this way. And he won't have to be assured in return that he is loved anyway. He will know it from past experience.

Children must also learn to cope with anger in others. There are times, of course, when children are especially irritating to adults (who don't lose their own capacity to be angry). After Father has twice explained that he's tired, and has asked Bobby to put off banging that drum until tomorrow, Bobby then learns from an impatient *"Put that thing away, NOW!"* that other people get angry. Of course the father who knows it's really his boss with whom he's vexed today tries not to take his feelings out on the children. But occasionally everyone does this sort of thing. As bewildering as anger without apparent reasons may be, children learn to understand and to cope with that, too, so long as it isn't constant or overwhelming.

An adult who trusts himself to show reasonable anger with children usually is freer to love them, just because the anger has not been tucked away somewhere. In exactly the same way, this applies to the child. If he has been free to vent his feelings of anger, he will more likely be able to express spontaneously his feelings of warmth and love. *See also* AGGRESSIVENESS; BITING; TEMPER TANTRUM.

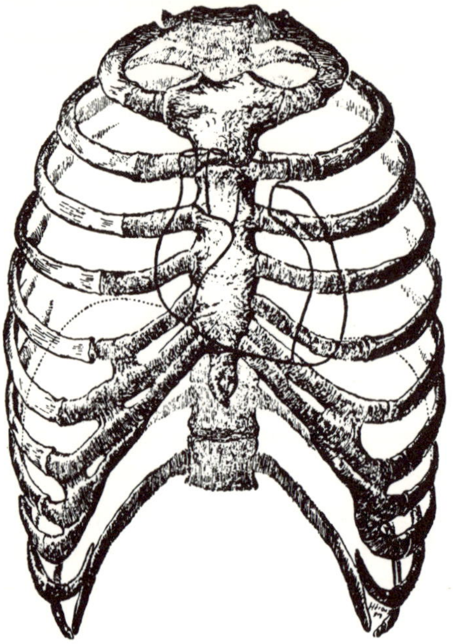

Angina Pectoris—The black outline shows the position of the heart in the chest cavity. The heart lies under the *sternum* (breastbone) and extends to the left of it. In the average-sized adult the heart weighs just under three-quarters of a pound.

ANGINA PECTORIS means pain in the chest, a symptom which accompanies any interference with blood supply or oxygenation of the heart muscle. Men are affected five times as often as women, and the symptom is seen most frequently in the sixth and seventh decades of life, though younger people are also affected. High-strung, sensitive, active people are most commonly subject to it, and in 90 per cent of cases, *arteriosclerosis,* or hardening of the arteries, is noted. Persons with diabetes, high blood pressure, rheumatic heart disease, and anemia are more susceptible than others to angina pectoris.

The heart muscles, like all muscles, depend upon the constant flow of oxygen-rich blood into the tissues in order to perform their required work and sustain their health. The blood vessels which supply the heart with blood are the coronary vessels. Any change in the caliber of these significant vessels, such as sudden narrowing or blockage, will seriously interfere with the flow of oxygen and nourishment to the heart muscle. When this occurs, pain results.

The pain of angina pectoris is typically brief, lasting seldom more than three or four minutes. When longer, the cause may be something else. The pain is just under the breastbone and often radiates to the neck and down the left arm. Occasionally it may move from the chest to the right arm, the stomach, or back.

In most persons, exertion or emotion precipitates the attack. Under these circumstances, the heart muscle beats more rapidly and needs a faster, richer supply of oxygen and blood. If the coronary vessels are partially blocked by fatty deposits, as in arteriosclerosis, the circulation is not able to cope with the increased demands by the heart and angina results. Angina frequently occurs after a heavy meal, because of the increased work load digestion places on the heart. A man who may be able to walk rapidly without distress at a time when he has no food in his stomach may be unable to walk even a hundred feet after he has had a heavy meal. The attack of angina pectoris is likely to occur following a meal which is eaten too hastily, in which case considerable air is taken in with the food. It may also follow a meal which is indigestible or eaten when one is too tired.

Any strong emotion may precipitate an attack of angina, especially grief, anger, or worry. It may also occur in any occupation, though less commonly to laborers because of their better muscular development. Angina pectoris is more prevalent in cities, probably because of the faster paced life associated with cities.

Moderation is of the utmost importance in controlling angina pectoris. At the first sign of chest pain, the person should immediately cease what he is doing and sit down and rest. Relief of pain will often come in a few minutes. To persist in exertion after the onset of pain is extremely hazardous, and in this respect the pain is a significant symptom which informs the patient that he is overexerting himself and needs rest.

Fortunately many drugs are available which give immediate relief to those with angina pectoris or a tendency to narrowing of the coronary vessels for whatever reason. Most popular is *nitroglycerine,* which causes a dilation, or widening, of the coronary vessels during an attack and thus permits more blood to flow through. Nitroglycerine, taken as a small tablet slipped under the tongue during an attack, brings relief almost immediately, and seldom later than two or three minutes. *Amylnitrate,* a medicine which is inhaled during an attack, can also be taken. Other drugs of a similar nature may be regularly prescribed for two or three times a day to prevent attacks. No drugs should be taken without consulting a doctor, as they may have unpleasant or serious side-effects.

Two drugs now used in the treatment of angina pectoris are *propanolol* (AYERST®, INDERAL®) and *isosorbide dinitrate* (ISORDIL®). Although undesirable side effects may appear when these drugs are taken separately, these reactions tend to be minimized when the drugs are taken together. Propanolol functions by blocking the sympathetic nervous system, slowing the heart beat and decreasing the requirement of the heart muscle. Isosorbide dinitrate dilates the coronary vessels so that more oxygen reaches the heart.

Relief of the acute attack, though momentarily significant, is not the entire solution to angina pectoris. The person's daily life must be reguated so as to avoid situations liable to affect adversely the circulation to the heart. Here are ten rules which are applicable to the person with angina pectoris:

1. Do not subject your heart to sudden, strenuous, or prolonged physical activity.
2. Eat regularly, slowly, and temperately.
3. Make every effort to keep your weight down, particularly after the

age of forty. Angina pectoris is many times more common and serious in overweight persons.

4. Avoid physical activity for at least thirty minutes after eating a heavy meal.

5. Avoid emotional stress and strain. Plan your work so that you get sufficient rest. Avoid worry.

6. Keep your body healthy and free from infection.

7. Avoid constipation.

8. Get at least eight hours of sleep a night in a room well supplied with fresh air.

9. Keep fit with a regular moderate program of exercise.

10. See your doctor regularly for a thorough checkup.

The person who suffers from angina pectoris should not despair of his situation. It is not a disease, but a warning of danger from the heart. It is quite possible to live a fairly normal existence if the person takes proper care of himself and always heeds the warning signal of pain. *See also* HEART; CIRCULATORY SYSTEM. *See* MEDIGRAPHS pages 697, 1273.

► Diseases of the Heart and Circulation, *Angina Pectoris,* 1299.

ANGINA, VINCENT'S. *See* VINCENT'S ANGINA.

ANILINE, a colorless, oily liquid prepared from coal tar or benzene or indigo, used extensively in numerous industries for the manufacture of various chemicals, among them acetanilid, acriflavine, methylene blue, and other antiseptic dyes. Aniline is highly poisonous and may enter the body through broken skin or through inhalation or ingestion of the oil or its fumes or dusts, and thus lead to poisoning of the body. Acute poisoning will cause sudden prostration; blue discoloration of the lips, nose, and fingers; and may be accompanied by unconsciousness and convulsions. In case of poisoning, the doctor should be called immediately and the patient kept warm and given an emetic of a tablespoon of mustard in a glass of water. *See also* POISONING.

ANIMAL BITES AND WOUNDS. Animal bites often present a danger of *rabies.* Warm-blooded animals such as dogs, cats, and wild mammals including bats may transmit rabies. First aid procedure calls for the immediate washing of the animal wound thoroughly and finding medical care at once. Rabies always is fatal if it develops but preventive medical measures are available. Don't kill the dog or cat unless essential. Confine it at a veterinary facility or humane society. Its symptoms then can be observed; if death ensues, the animal's head can be examined for evidence of rabies. Should the animal be killed at once, the findings may not be clear. If the animal must be killed, do not injure the brain and thereby interfere with laboratory examination of the head.

Wounds from venomous animals are of another sort. Restrict activity at once if bitten by a *venomous snake.* Quickly wrap a constriction band around the limb just above the bite. Make a few longitudinal cuts through the skin at points where the poison most likely is deposited. Crosscuts intersecting the longitudinal ones should not be deep lest tendons be severed. Then apply suction with the mouth or a suction cup during transport to a medical facility. Ice applications interspersed with the suction may help. Keep the limb lowered. For the sting of a *venomous scorpion,* wrap a constriction band around the affected part, usually a finger, for five minutes and then release it. Meanwhile apply ice, continuing until medical help is obtained. *Tarantulas* of this country are not venomous; imported ones may be. First aid for bites by the venomous ones and by *black widow spiders* is the same as for poisonous scorpions. In case of *bee sting,* remove the poison sac with a tweezers without emptying it into the tissue—for these injuries as well as for the bites or stings of mosquitoes, chiggers, and the like, palliative measures include the application of ammonia water, cold cream, or baking-soda paste. Immediate application of ice gives much relief. Good insect repellents are available too. *See also* RABIES; RAT-BITE FEVER; TULAREMIA; BEE STINGS; INSECT BITES; SNAKEBITE.

ANIMALS, FEAR OF. In dealing with a youngster's fears of animals—as with others fears—it is important to distinguish between real and imagined ones. It is not unrealistic for a youngster, for instance, to hesitate about patting a strange dog when he doesn't know how friendly or unfriendly it may be. It is quite natural for children to be afraid of a new or large or over-exuberant animal. It's usually not difficult to reassure a child in these fairly common situations and to see to it that he is reasonably cautious but at the same time is not denied enjoyable experiences with safe animals. In trying to get young children used to animals, it's generally best to start with small animals—a kitten, a puppy, or a rabbit. If the adult holds it and pats it, the child will probably begin to make tentative gestures toward it and gradually overcome his timidity and be ready for a closer approach.

Sometimes adults make children too cautious because of their own fears. A mother who cannot bear to have her son put his face near a kitten's fur, another who shrinks when her little girl picks up a bug—these mothers are not apt to have children who will feel friendly to animals. Children sense feelings too well for adults to try to conceal their fears completely. But children *can* understand also that some people enjoy some things and other people don't. A statement like "Yes, that's a nice collie, but I don't like dogs very much. You do, I know, so go ahead and pat him," is, to a youngster, usually quite understandable.

A fear of animals that has no basis in reality is harder to deal with, of course. A boy or girl who loves an enormous Irish setter, for example, may be terrified of a tiny kitten. Such fears seldom have anything to do with the animal in question but probably represent something altogether different. At times the fear of an animal is an indication that a child has been upset by some past event in his life—moving to a new home, going to a hospital, or separation from his parents. Or at times a child may be disturbed by more general feelings of not measuring up to what his parents expect of him, or feeling guilty over some "bad" thing he has done or thought. He may then fear that the punishment he deserves will come in the form of being hurt by an animal.

Though it is difficult to determine the specific causes of a child's fear, there are at least some definite measures that should be avoided. To force the child to come near or touch the animal will not remove this fear and may more likely increase his terror. A youngster needs instead to be reassured that his fear is nothing to be ashamed of, that many children feel the same, and that he will eventually get over it himself. He needs to feel the love and support of his parents when he is frightened. If the child is willing, it occasionally helps for a protecting adult to approach the animal with him. Any suggestion of forcing, however, any insistence that it is important to overcome the fear immediately, will only prolong it. And the more successful a child feels his general achievements and activities are, the more self-assurance he can bring to conquering his fear of animals.

ANISEIKONIA. There are many strange Latin names that describe disturbances of vision due to changes from the normal in the shape of either the eyeball or the mechanism that brings the image through to the brain. For instance *astigmatism* is a condition in which parallel rays are focused at different points and is usually due to a change in the curvature of the cornea, or outside of the eye.

There is another condition in which there is marked inequality in the refraction of the two eyes. This occurs in a person who is farsighted in one eye and nearsighted in the other eye. Sometimes either farsightedness or nearsightedness is combined with astigmatism.

One of the most recently discovered conditions is one in which the images which fall on the retina in back of the eye are unequal in either size or shape. This condition is called *aniseikonia.* There are apparently instances in which such inequality in the retinal images is responsible for eyestrain and in which correction of the refraction or the wearing of suitable glasses does not bring complete relief.

Instruments have been developed to test the ability of a person to see images equally with either eye. A person with aniseikonia will think that a table is level when it is actually tipped or vice versa. If a table is level and looks tipped, the person can be asked to tip the table until it seems level to him. The amount of tipping necessary to make the table seem level will give an idea of the amount of distortion present.

Eye specialists say that about 2 per cent of people have aniseikonia that can be corrected. About one third of all the people who are given glasses to correct this condition report that they are entirely relieved of the symptoms; another one third say that they have partial relief.

While the correction of aniseikonia will not clear up headaches, which may be the result of many different causes, there are instances of headache in which correction of this solution will bring about some relief. *See also* EYE.

ANKLE, a joint between the leg and the foot, formed by the junction of the lower ends of the *tibia* and *fibula,* the bones of the lower leg, and the *astragalus,* or anklebone, in the foot.

Sprained ankle. Sudden twisting of the foot may stretch one of the many ligaments which connect various bones in the ankle area, and produce local bleeding, swelling, and extreme tenderness. Immediate application of cold compresses is helpful to reduce swelling, bleeding, and pain during the first twenty-four hours. Strapping the ankle with elastic bandages or adhesive tape relieves tension and mobility of the joint and hastens healing. Daily submersion in hot water and rest are also beneficial and soothing. The latest treatment includes injection of *novocaine* solutions for relief of pain, as well as *hyaluronidase* to decrease swelling, to permit earlier use of the foot.

Painful ankle. A painful ankle may occur with a sprain, fracture of ankle bones, arthritis, or gout.

Swollen ankle. Swollen ankle may occur in many conditions, especially in pregnancy, kidney disease, heart disease, and in overweight persons, because of impaired circulation. Many persons, women especially, develop swollen ankles in hot weather. *See also* JOINTS AND JOINT DISORDERS; SPRAINS.

ANODYNE, any agent that will relieve pain. *See also* ANALGESIA; ANESTHESIA.

ANOREXIA, the scientific term for loss of appetite.

ANOREXIA NERVOSA, a condition most frequently found in young neurotic women, characterized by a pronounced aversion to food, due to a hysterical condition. In extreme cases, the loss of weight may be so great that death may ensue if the malady is not corrected in time. Both psychological and medical treatment are necessary.

ANOSMIA, complete loss of the sense of smell. It may be permanent or temporary, depending on whether or not the olfactory nerves are damaged or destroyed completely beyond hope of healing. Partial loss of the sense of smell is *hyposmia,* and the loss of smell in one nostril only is *hemianosmia.* An excessive response to odors is known as *hyperosmia.*

Loss of the sense of smell may be the result of a mental state, as in hysteria. In some instances of hallucination, the person imagines that he smells certain odors not actually present. Treatment of anosmia due to mental causes is difficult.

Defects of the sense of smell may be caused by dryness of the mucous membranes of the nose, by infection, injury, obstruction, deterioration of the nasal tissue, or by action of drugs. Certain diseases of the brain, brain injury, or brain tumor may also produce anosmia.

Tests to determine the presence of a sense of smell are made by releasing certain odors and noting the responses. Adjustment to the loss of a sense of smell is usually not too difficult. *See also* OLFACTORY SENSE.

ANOXEMIA, a lack of the normal amount of oxygen in the blood, due to high altitudes, low partial pressure of oxygen in anesthesia, cardiac failure, or strangling.

ANTABUSE, a drug used in the treatment of alcoholics to produce a distaste for alcohol. When antabuse is administered to an alcoholic, extreme discomfort, severe nausea, vomiting, and flushing develop, with intolerance to alcohol.

Antabuse should never be given to a person who is intoxicated, nor should it be given without the full knowledge and consent of the person. The drug is best used in conjunction with psychotherapy. *See also* ALCOHOLISM.

ANTACID, a substance that relieves acidity and neutralizes acids.

ANTENATAL denotes the time from conception to delivery.

ANTEPARTUM refers to any occurrence or condition that takes place before the baby is born.

ANTHRAX, a malignant carbuncle, is a serious infectious disease which not only attacks animals such as cattle and sheep but is also transmitted by them to human beings. The germ, found most often in the recently ejected excrement of animals or men, or in their hair or skin, is transmitted to or may enter the body through a wound, scratch, or insect bite, or through inhalation. The most frequent victims of anthrax are farmers, butchers, veterinarians, and hide workers. Anthrax of the lung is often referred to as "wool sorters' disease."

The prevention of anthrax among human beings is best achieved by protecting the animals. Failing this, obvious precautions are necessary, especially in places where men work with animals or with the products of animals. Clothing, such as overalls and rubber aprons, which protects the skin should be worn. Persons sorting hair or wool should wear breathing devices which will protect them from the inhalation of dangerous substances. Workers are advised to cleanse their hands with disinfectants when their work is done. Some precautions are merely those which any efficient industrial management insists upon: general sanitation, attention to skin lesions of workers, disinfection of dangerous wastage before it leaves the factory, and effective ventilation. Exhaust fans are particularly essential to carry away any dangerous substances which might exist in the atmosphere.

The first symptom of anthrax is painful itching. Several hours later, somewhere on the body, an inflamed pimple or boil develops which becomes hard, has a purple center, and is surrounded by a zone of red. As the boil swells, it produces a thick and bloody pus at its center, and at the same time the adjacent lymph glands swell and the veins become inflamed. The first boil is followed by many others. Eventually gangrene may develop in the infected tissue. Simultaneously the person is likely to suffer from a general weakness, together with chilliness, disinclination to eat, nausea, and a high temperature. The most serious form of this disease is anthrax of the lungs.

Serums have been developed which are useful against this malady. The sulfa drugs and other antibiotics have also been valuable, especially in the control of supplementary infections. Unfortunately, because of the rarity of the disease, the diagnosis sometimes is made too late to counteract the infection and save the patient. *See also* OCCUPATIONAL DISEASES, BIOLOGICAL HAZARDS.

ANTIBIOTICS, substances produced during the growth of molds or bacteria which inhibit or kill other bacteria that cause disease.

The search for effective and nontoxic antibiotics is unceasing. Molds and bacteria are grown and examined for antibiotic substances by bacteriologists and mycologists. Chemists then purify these substances and prepare them as concentrates which in turn are tested in animal experiments by pathologists to determine their potency and toxicity before they can be employed for human use.

Since the development of penicillin in 1942, following its accidental discovery in 1929 during an experiment by Sir Alexander Fleming, the English bacteriologist, thousands of antibiotic substances have been isolated and studied. About twenty of these are now in active use, and a detailed description of the leading ones follows.

A new antibiotic drug *erythromycin* was developed from a fungus growth found in a sample of soil collected in the Philippines. The brand name of this product is *Ilotycin.* It has minimal effects on the digestive tract and is capable of attacking a wide range of organisms.

Bacitracin was one of the earlier discovered antibiotics; it destroys a wide variety of germs such as the *streptococci,* the *pneumococci,* the *gonococci,* and the *meningococci.* The drug is not taken by mouth to the extent that others are.

Magnamycin is known also as *carbomycin.* This antibiotic was isolated from *Streptomyces halstedii.* It also inhibits the growth of a variety of organisms like the streptococci, staphylococci, and pneumococci.

Chloramphenacol is known as *chloromycetin.* This antibiotic is also derived from a form of streptomyces found in Venezuela. It is effective against certain gram negative organisms and against the germs known as *rickettsia.* This product has been more effective than others in the treatment of typhoid fever.

Chlortetracycline is the scientific name for the golden yellow antibiotic known as *aureomycin.* It has a wide variety of effectiveness against many organisms and occasionally has been considered effective against some virus conditions. This antibiotic has been used against Rocky Mountain spotted fever, typhus, scrub typhus, Q fever and Brill's disease; also against atypical pneumonia, psittacosis, or parrot fever. The antibiotic has been used against many forms of urinary tract infections and against infections by such organisms as those of anthrax, tularemia and actinomycosis. The antibiotic has been reported effective against amebic infections and acute intestinal infections. Aureomycin has been used in certain stages of syphilis in which it compares well with penicillin. Thus this antibiotic has been considered one of the most effective of all of this group.

Neomycin is an antibacterial substance derived from another streptomyces isolated by Waxman and known as the *Streptomyces fradiae.* This is used particularly in direct application in the form of ointments for various infections of the skin and eye, in the treatment of wounds, burns and ulcers, sties and other infections of the skin and hair follicle. The drug is used also as an intestinal antiseptic for destroying bacteria which are in the colon when there is to be surgery of the abdominal organs.

Oxytetracycline is more widely known as *terramycin.* It may stop the growth of various bacteria or destroy them and is widely used against the germs of the type of the streptococci, staphylococci, pneumococci and the organisms of influenza. It has been found effective in treating Rock Mountain spotted fever, typhus, Q fever and many conditions caused by rickettsia. The drug has been used for intestinal infections, amebic infections, pin worm infestation, gonorrhea and in certain stages of syphilis. These are only a few of the many uses of terramycin which physicians use in general almost as frequently as penicillin.

Benzathine penicillin G is a complex salt of penicillin which can be given by mouth or by injection and which has the advantage of continuing to act over a long period of time. Thus a single dose of 600,000 units may be injected into the muscles as a preventive measure a day before the removal of the tonsils, extraction of teeth or for various other minor surgical procedures. The drug is also used to prevent relapses in rheumatic fever or in congenital heart disease, and for eliminating streptococci in the human body. Especially valuable has been the use of this drug in the treatment of gonorrhea and syphilis.

Polymyxin is a term which designates a series of related antibiotics derived from certain bacteria found in soil. This antibiotic also attacks certain types of microorganisms, some of which have not been reached by penicillin or other antibiotics that have been mentioned. Its use for instance against influenza, certain forms of pneumonia and infections with bacillus Proteus makes it most worthwhile.

The principal use of *streptomycin* has been against the organisms of tuberculosis but it can also attack other infectious organisms. The physician determines by other laboratory studies which is the most effective antibiotic against the type of organism that affects his patient.

Tetracycline is almost known as *tetracyn.* This antibiotic also is isolated from certain streptomyces. It has actions and uses similar to those of chlortetracycline and oxytetracycline.

Viomycin is an antibiotic derived from *Streptomyces puniceus.* This is also an antituberculosis agent and has been used when the germs in certain patients have failed to respond to treatment with other antibiotics to which they have become insensitive.

In the use of the antibiotic drugs, physicians may use one or a mixture. These drugs have brought about an entirely new era in the control of infections so that many conditions which formerly threatened life are now either disappearing or have become innocuous.

In some countries all sorts of substances are being studied as to the possibility of producing new antibiotics. These are being derived from tomatoes, radishes, organisms found in soil, in fact from some germs themselves, such as the *bacillus subtilis,* which may yield substances that are antibiotic for other germs.

New in the use of antibiotics is employment of a combination of *nystatin,* an antifungal antibiotic, with tetracycline in the treatment of a number of conditions. The advantage of such a mixture is said to be its ability to prevent the invasion of various fungi following elimination of bacteria by antibiotics. Investigators reported that a combination of oxytetracycline and neomycin antibiotics did not prevent fungal overgrowth but that the combination was effective in eradicating proteus organisms as invaders. Studies were made on the combination of nystatin

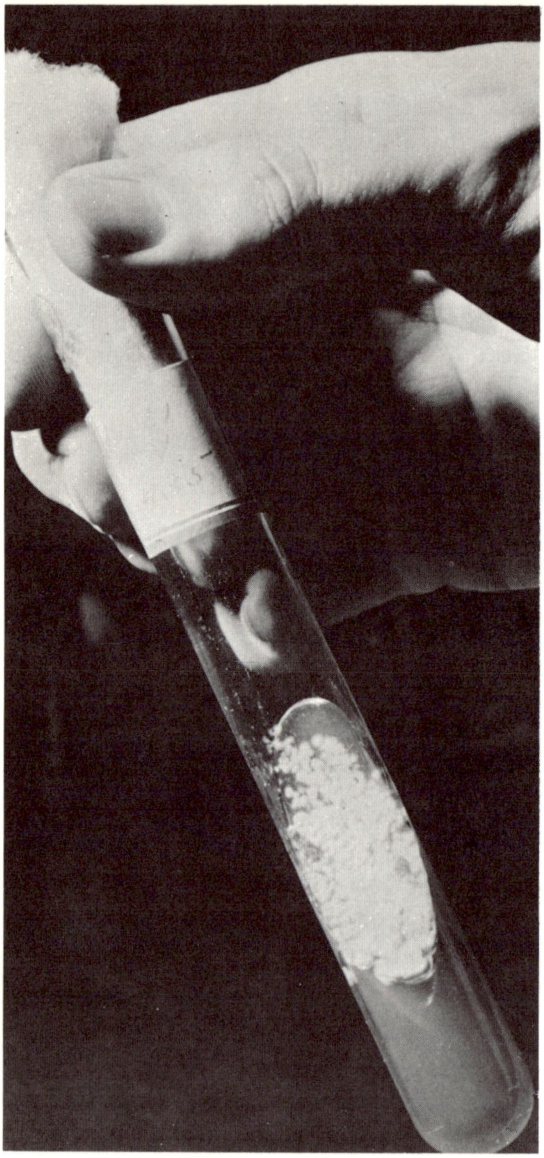

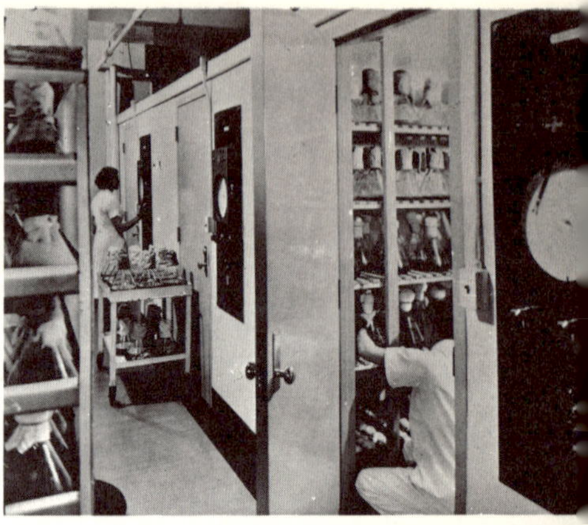

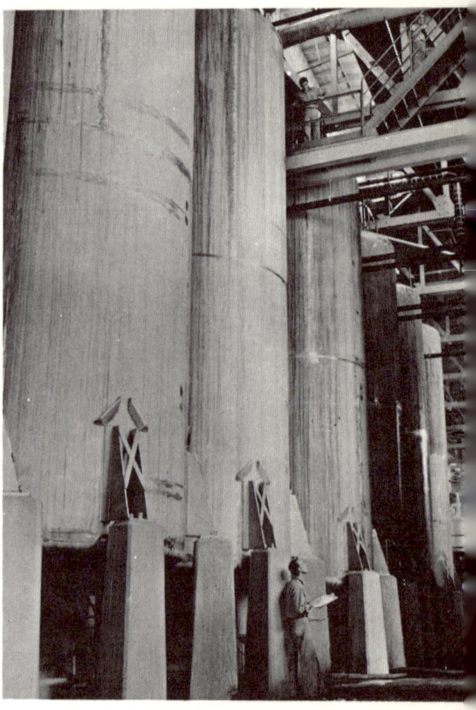

The development of antibiotics has been one of the most remarkable accomplishments of the twentieth century. Having begun in 1929 with penicillin, the list of these miracle drugs is now growing with extraordinary rapidity. Streptomycin, aureomycin, chloromycetin, erythromycin, bacitracin, carbomycin, neomycin, terramycin, tetracyn, polymixin, nystatin, isoniazid, and ethambutol are some of the chemicals being used with excellent results in the combat against such scourges as tuberculosis, pneumonia, syphilis, gonorrhea, chancroid, tularemia, anthrax, septic sore throat, and other diseases caused by bacterial organisms. The antibiotics are also effective against rickettsial organisms causing such diseases as typhus, scrub typhus, and Rocky Mountain spotted fever. They have been used successfully against certain parasitic diseases, such as amebic dysentery, and against some fungus diseases, such as actinomycosis. However, only a few viruses have responded to antibiotic treatment.

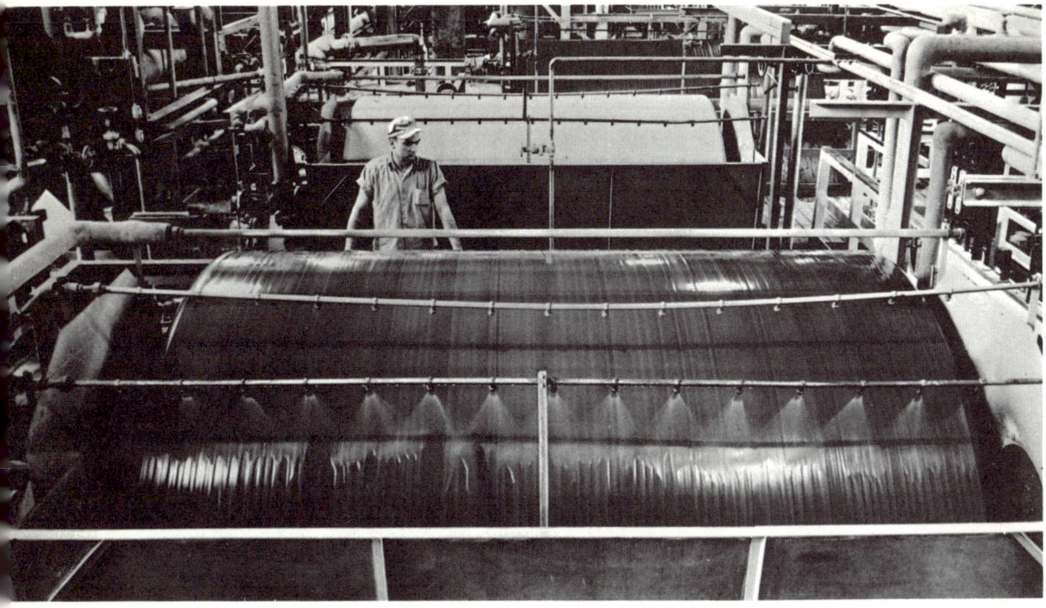

Antibiotics are derived from molds. The molds are grown in a nutrient medium, such as can be seen in the test tube shown in the left-hand photograph *(opposite page)*. From the original nutrient medium in the test tube, the mold is transferred to other nutrient media in large incubators where a fermentation process occurs. This fermentation process is continued subsequently in large antiseptic tanks. Incubators can be seen in the upper right-hand photograph *(opposite page)*, and the tanks below. Even the air in the tanks is sterilized. The mold is separated from the liquid nutrient medium in a rotary vacuum filter *(above)*. It may take a million pints of liquid to produce a hundred pounds of antibiotic. The antibiotic is converted into an insoluble salt and removed by filtration *(below, left)*. The crude antibiotic salt must go through several stages of purification. It is redissolved and converted to crystals. The crystals are collected and dried in a vacuum *(below, right)*. The crystals are then dissolved again and the solution passed through fine filters to entrap bacteria.

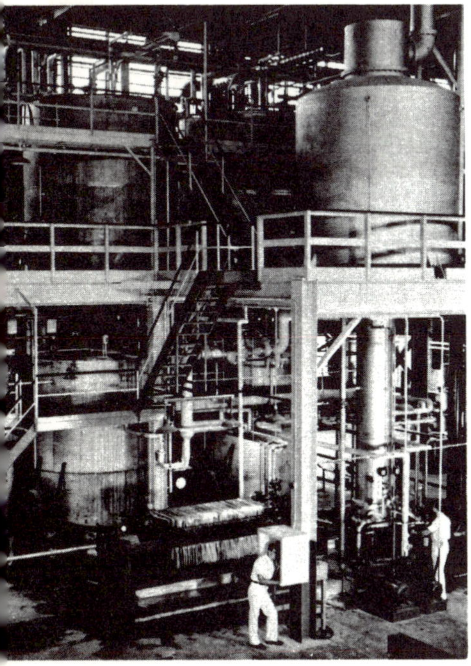

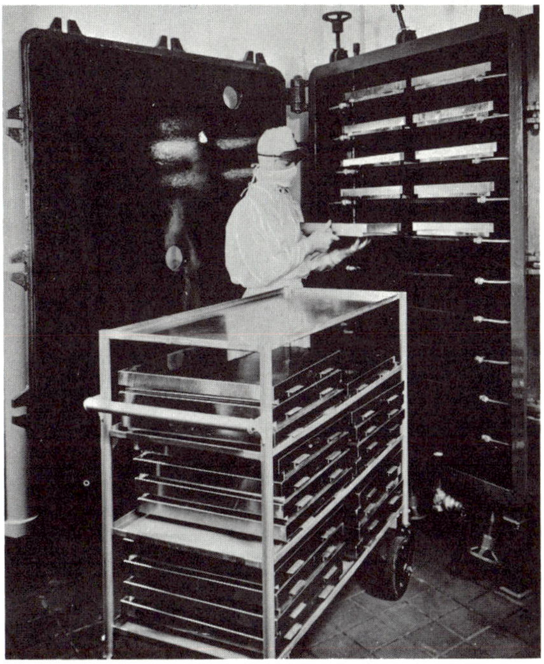

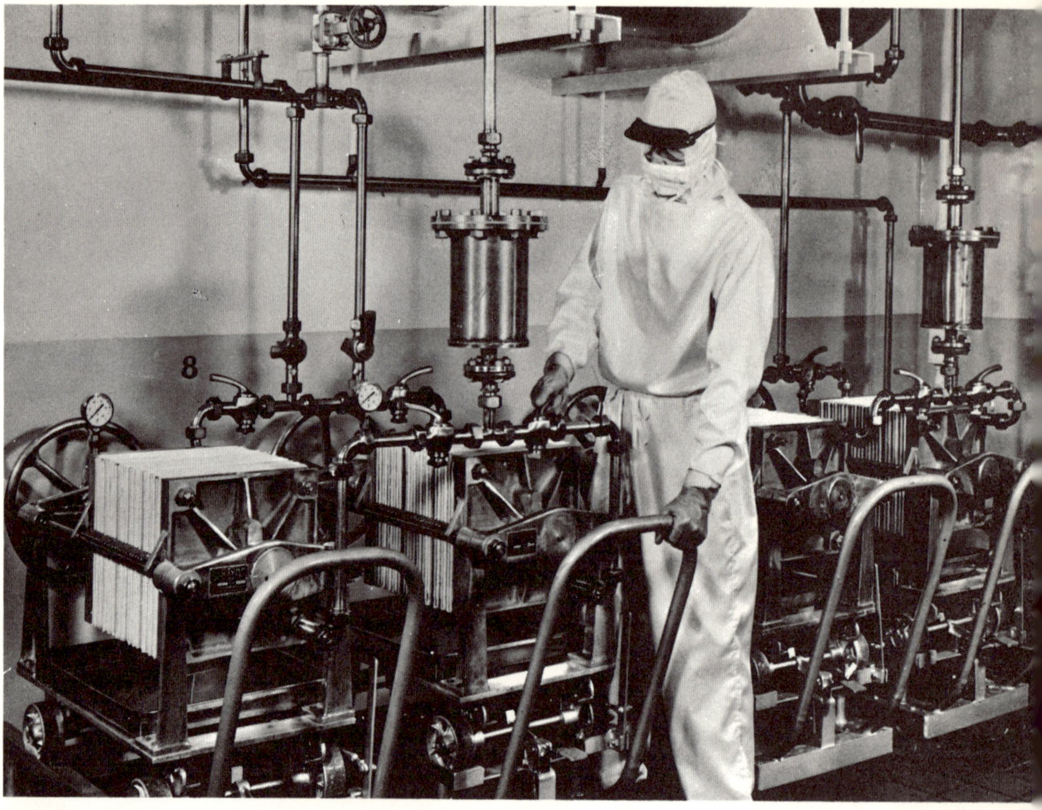

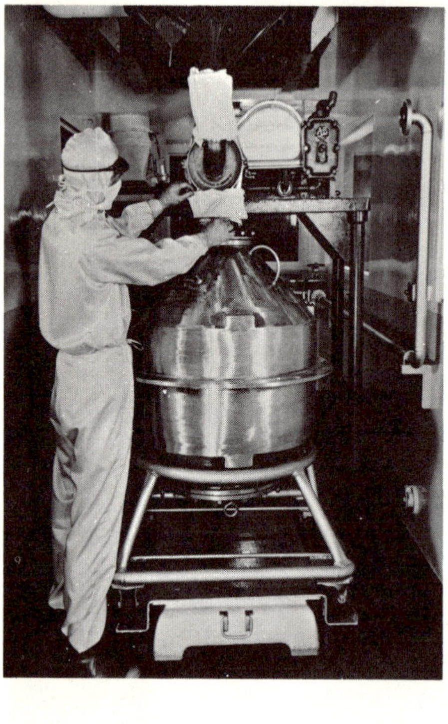

The filtering mechanism to remove bacteria is shown above. After recrystallization, the antibiotic is dried and ground. Bottling and packaging are important steps in the preparation of antibiotics. These procedures must be performed under scrupulously antiseptic conditions. The upper left-hand photograph on the opposite page shows bottles being greatly magnified for a rigid visual inspection. In the upper right-hand photograph, antibiotics are being deposited in inspected bottles. Below, further inspection takes place. Every possible precaution is taken to prevent contamination, and manufacturing facilities are regularly inspected by government officials. Samples from each batch of antibiotic are taken at every stage of the manufacturing process. These samples are analyzed in the control laboratory to ensure the purity of the shipment. Antibiotics inhibit the growth of a wide variety of organisms, such as the streptococci, staphylococci, and pneumococci. Their principal deficiency is ineffectiveness against most virus diseases.

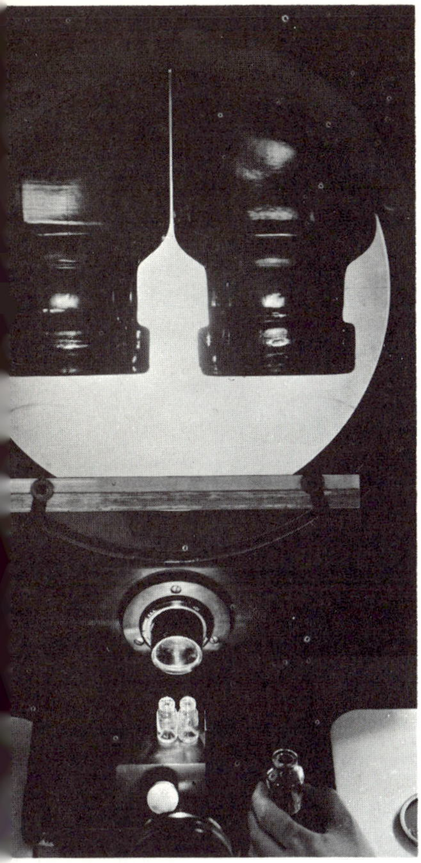

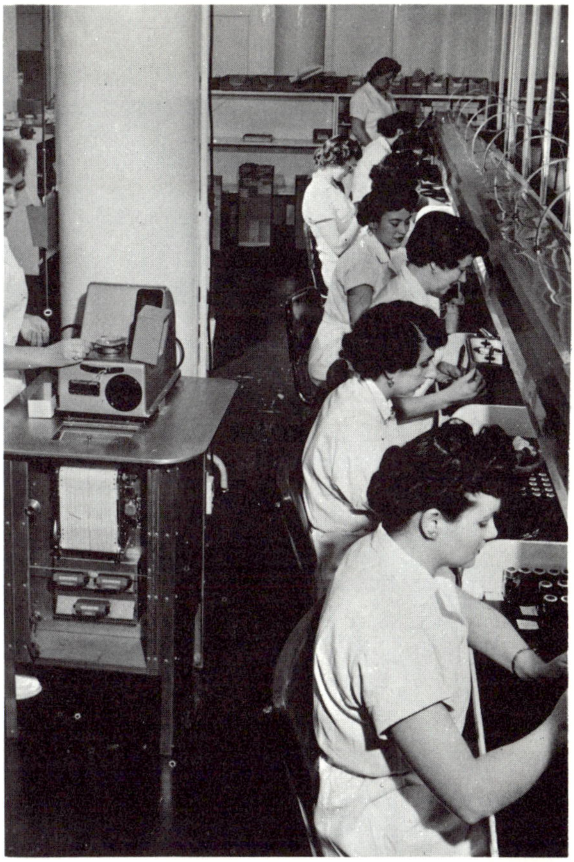

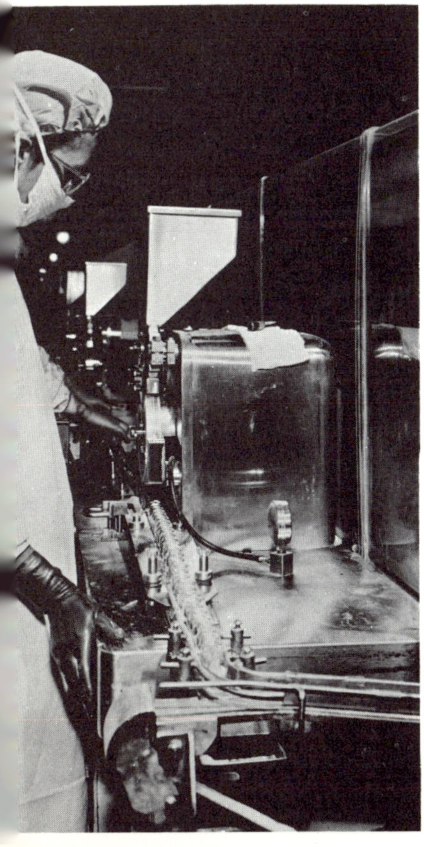

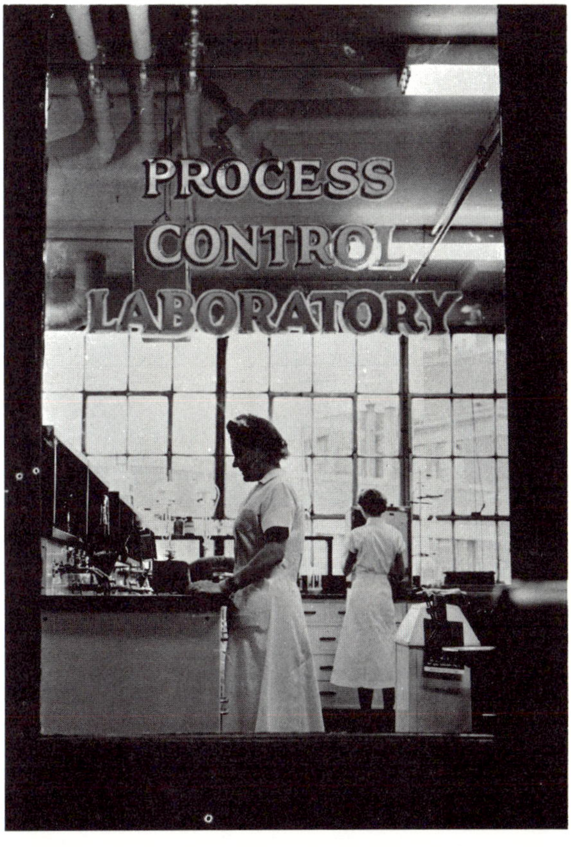
PROCESS
CONTROL
LABORATORY

and tetracycline and found effective in a variety of bacterial infections.

Among the thousands of substances now under investigation physicians expect to develop some which will be able to attack the viruses of diseases like poliomyelitis and encephalitis as well as other conditions heretofore not amenable to treatment.

In some instances, antibiotics have produced undesirable reactions, such as diarrhea, nausea, vomiting, and abdominal cramps, and may also cause serious damage to the kidneys or other organs. When used indiscriminately, antibiotics may lead to growth within the body of new strains of previously harmless bacteria which become drug-resistant and thus expose the patient to residual infections. Most doctors believe that antibiotics should not be used in conditions, such as minor colds and sore throats, which are readily controlled by simple remedies. The patient's response to antibiotics should not be endangered or his immunity to disease decreased by the use of antibiotics for minor infections. *See also* SULFONAMIDE DRUGS; IMMUNIZATION; VACCINATION; ANTITOXIN; ANTIHISTAMINIC DRUGS; BACTERIA; VIRUSES; ANTIBODY; ANTIMALARIAL DRUGS; BACTERIAL ENDOCARDITIS; MEDICINE CHEST; PNEUMONIA.

► Drugs and Their Uses, *Antibiotics,* 902.

ANTIBODY, a substance, natural or artificial, introduced to serve as a protection against infections or foreign proteins in the body fluids. Antagonistic to factors which are injurious to the animal organisms, an antibody can destroy bacteria adequately and counteract poisons that cause infections. *See also* ANTITOXIN; BLOOD TYPES; GAMMA GLOBULIN.

ANTICOAGULANT, a substance or condition which opposes or prevents coagulation or clotting. *See also* COAGULATION.

ANTIDOTE, any agent used to prevent or to counteract the effect of a poison. There are specific antidotes for different poisons; for a full discussion, *see* POISONING.

ANTIFEBRIN, or *acetanilid,* a drug derived from aniline by the action of acetic acid upon it. Antifebrin has been used to lower fever, but more often serves to relieve pain and is therefore one of the ingredients frequently found in headache remedies. *See also* ACETANILID.

ANTIHISTAMINIC DRUGS, synthetic substances, used to alleviate allergic conditions by diminishing the action of *histamine.* Histamine is normally found in the body but in allergic conditions is liberated in excess. There are at least 25 antihistaminic drugs on the market. They come in tablets, solutions, sprays, eye drops, nose drops and ointments. They appear in mixtures for colds, cough, skin eruptions, and

The Eye—Organ of Sight

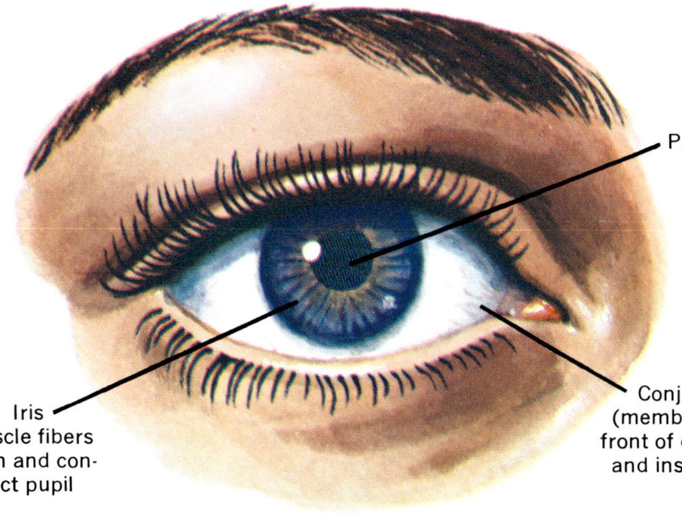

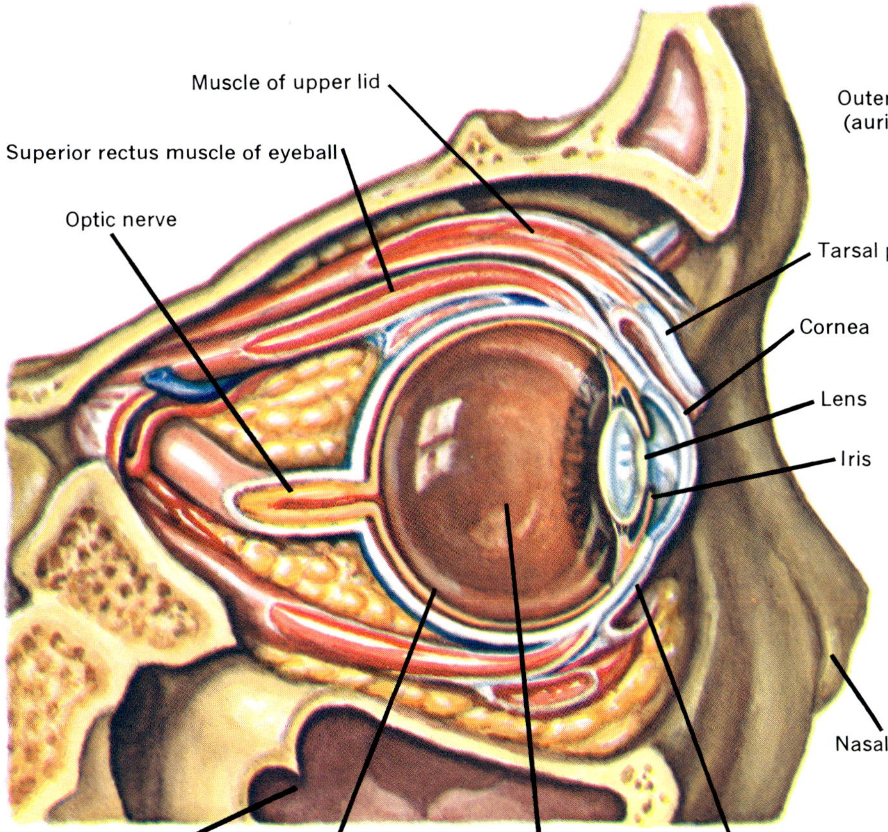

SIDE VIEW OF EYEBALL IN BONY ORBIT OR SOCKET

The Ear—Organ of Hearing

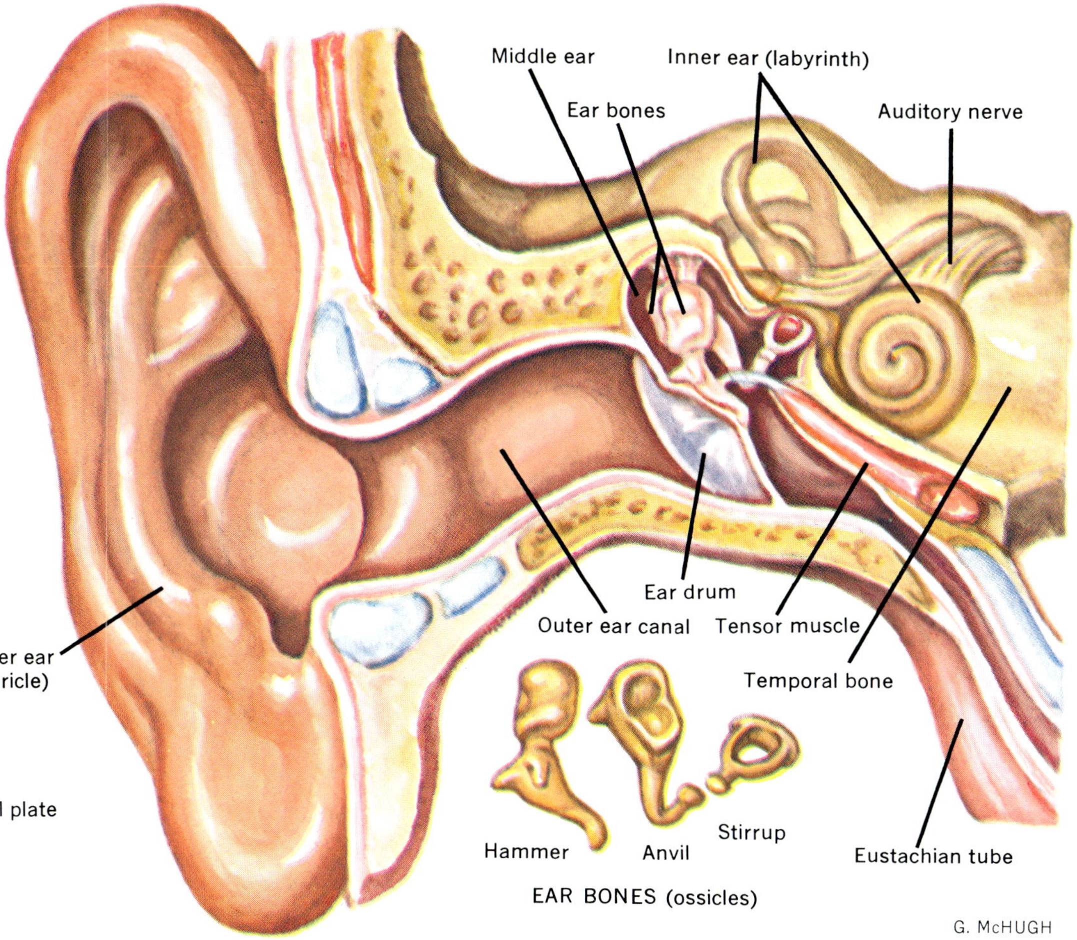

EAR BONES (ossicles)

THE INNER EAR, a series of fluid-filled channels in the temporal bone is an organ of both hearing and balance. In the hearing part, or cochlea, the membranous labyrinth (shown in blue) contains free hairy endings of the auditory nerve.

When sound waves collected by the outer ear vibrate the ear drum it sets the ossicles in motion. The stirrup pushing through the oval window bulges out the round window membrane and sets the fluid in motion. The waving auditory hairs send messages to the brain and the vibrations are identified and "heard". G. McH.

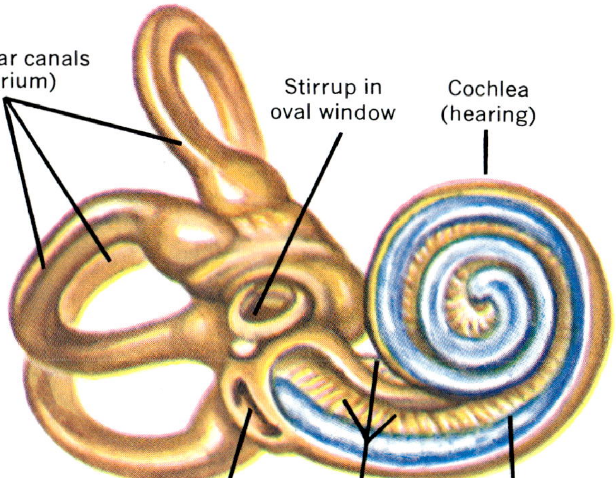

THE INNER EAR OR LABYRINTH

THE SPECIAL SENSE ORGANS

of Sight, Hearing, Smell and Taste

The special sense organs are really extensions of the brain—its external receptors—which report on the world around us.* In man, the most highly specialized organs are the eye and the ear; in many of the lower animals smell is the dominant sensory organ.

*For the brain areas that interpret these sensations, see "Functional Map of the Brain", Vol. 12.

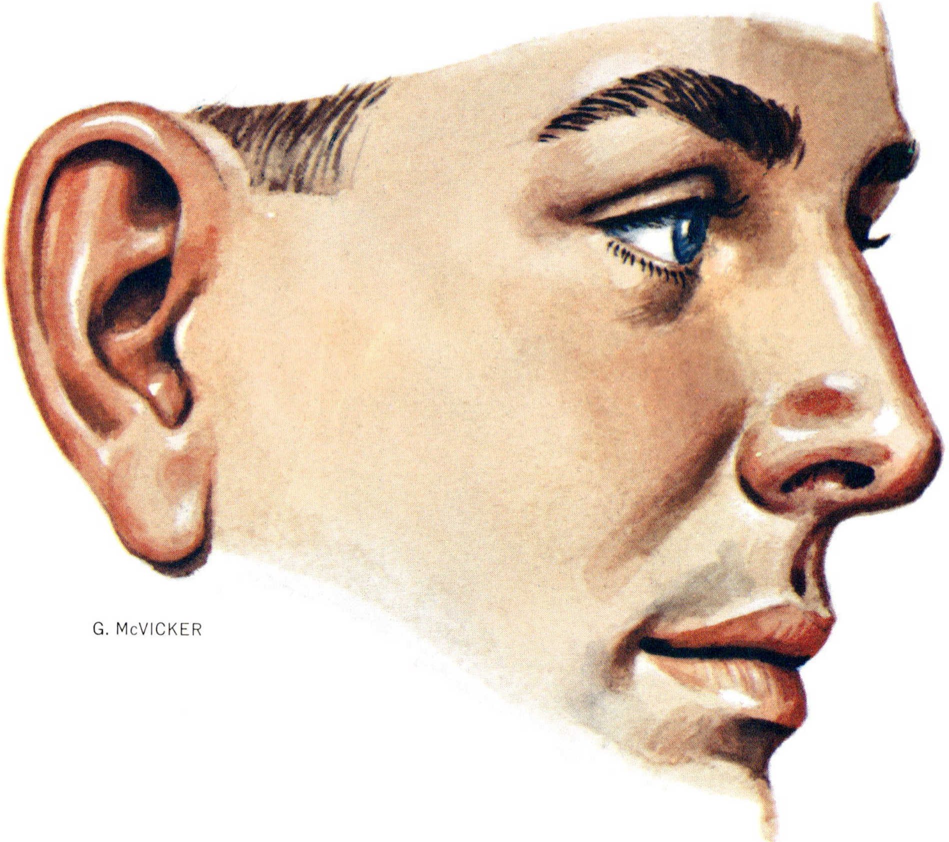

The external aspect of the organs of the special senses reveal nothing of the elaborate nerve apparatus within them. Only the openings through which stimuli reach the nerve receptors are visible—pupil of the eye, ear canal, nostrils and mouth.

The Organs of Smell and Taste

The smell region of the nose is in the upper part of the two nasal cavities. The taste areas of the mouth are most concentrated on the tongue, where taste buds cluster around the papillae. There are four kinds, reporting sweet, salty, acid (sour) and bitter tastes. Smell somewhat affects taste.

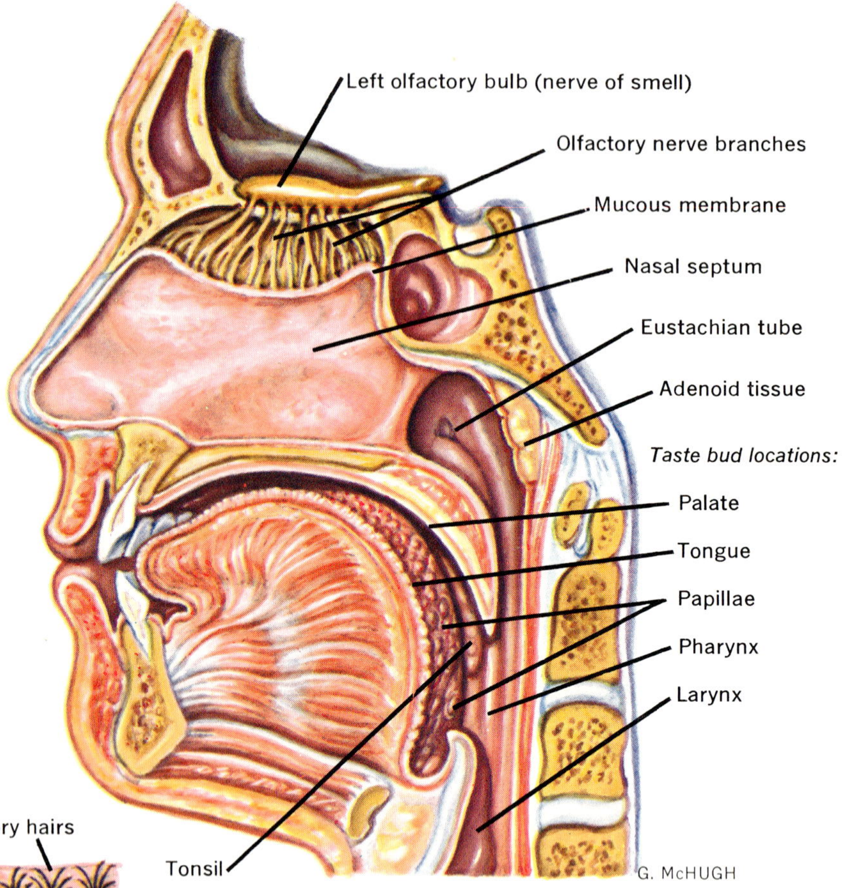

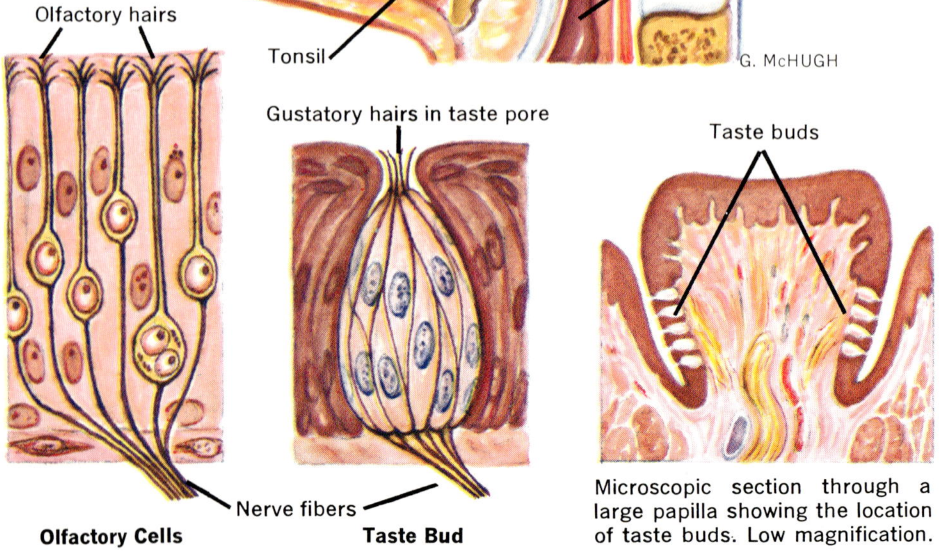

Microscopic section through a large papilla showing the location of taste buds. Low magnification.

NERVE RECEPTORS IN THE MUCOUS MEMBRANE

asthma. The most widely known are ANAHIST or NEOHETRAMINE which is *thonzylamine hydrochloride;* BENADRYL which is *diphenhydramine hydrochloride;* CHLORTRIMETON which is *chlorprophenpyridamine maleate;* MAREZINE which is *cyclizine hydrochloride;* PYRIBENZAMINE which is *tripelenamine hydrochloride;* and THEPHORIN which is *phenindamine tartrate.*

The claim that colds can be avoided by taking antihistamines shortly after the appearance of the first symptoms of a cold has not as yet been scientifically established. However, in combination with *aspirin* or *phenacetin,* or sprayed into the nose with *camphor,* antihistaminic preparations are useful in treating colds which begin with a running nose due to allergy. They also may relieve stuffiness, irritated eyes, and similar symptoms. Two of these preparations, available without a prescription, are TRIAMINICIN® and SINUTAB®.

Antihistaminic drugs are not a cure; they may obscure the real symptoms and are occasionally harmful. *See also* ALLERGY; SINUSES. *See* MEDIGRAPH page 2087.

► Drugs and Their Uses, *Antihistamines,* 900.

ANTI-HYPERTENSIVES. Many drugs have been introduced in recent years which aid physicians in treating patients with *hypertension* or high blood pressure and *arteriosclerosis* or hardening of the arteries. Obviously the choice of the remedy must rest with the physician who has studied his patient.

Among the most effective of drugs recently introduced is *hexamethonium tartrate.* The drug is available in many different preparations. The drug acts by blocking the nerve influences on the kidney.

Two drugs derived from *veratrum* are known as *protoveratrine.* These drugs have been used for the treatment of *essential hypertension* and *malignant hypertension;* in fact, for almost all varieties of hypertension. They slow the heart rate and their use is usually followed by a fall in blood pressure. Among the drugs also used in hypertension is *rauwolfia* which has been used in India for many years. Sometimes rauwolfia is combined with other drugs, particularly sedatives which act on the nervous system and thus bring about a lowering in blood pressure.

Two new products include *hydralazine* which is known as APRESOLINE and *pentapyrrolidium* known as ANSOLYSEN. The latter is considered to be five times stronger than hexamethonium. This drug produces reduction in blood pressure but there are dangerous side effects which the physician must watch carefully.

ANTIMALARIAL DRUGS. Malaria is not important in the United States as either an endemic or epidemic disease. But throughout the world, it probably ranks high among the most important health and medical problems. Malaria is controlled by eliminating conditions favorable to the growth of the mosquitoes which spread the disease. For years physicians have known that *quinine* from the cinchona bark could control malaria. During World War II *atabrine* was developed as a synthetic capable of reaching the *plasmodium* that causes malaria. Since World War II many investigators have tried to find drugs which would attack the *plasmodium vivax* and eliminate it from the body. During the war two new compounds called *chloraquine* and *paludrine* were developed which could prevent and cure malignant *tertian malaria* but which were only suppressive for *benign tertian malaria.* More recently a new derivative called *primaquine* has been found capable of preventing the relapses of malaria which have been produced in volunteers by bites of mosquitoes infected with *plasmodium vivax.* Also a pyrimidine derivative named *daraprim* has been found and is recognized as one of the most important antimalarial drugs. Daraprim was tried in a village in the Congo and after being given weekly to all the inhabitants for eleven weeks, reduced the incidence of malarial parasites in the blood from 22 per cent to zero.

ANTIMONY, a metallic crystalline substance, symbolized by *Sb* from the ancient word *stibium,* present in many minerals. It is extensively used in the manufacture of alloy metals.

Formerly a mainstay in medical practice, salts of antimony are now less frequently used. They diminish the functional activity of the heart and the arteries, in which case they act as depressants; they increase perspiration, (as diaphoretics), and they induce vomiting, (as emetics).

Antimony is effective in cases of infestation by flukes, which are flat parasitic worms.

ANTISEPTICS, substances that hinder the growth and activity of microorganisms, or germs. Antiseptic agents differ from those which act as disinfectants, germicides, or deodorants. A disinfectant or germicide kills bacteria which cause infectious diseases; a deodorant destroys or covers disagreeable odors. Substances like *chloride of lime* can be used for either purpose.

In surgery, the use of antiseptics is essential, especially in disinfecting instruments and other materials used in operations. In first aid for accidental wounds and in the care of contaminated or suppurating wounds, antiseptics prevent infection from spreading in the body.

Various antiseptics may be used to disinfect a wound. *Tincture of iodine* is recommended in first aid. Antiseptic dyes, like *tincture of merthiolate,* that can be painted on cuts and wounds are as powerful as iodine and less likely to burn or damage living tissue. Other antiseptics include *Mercurochrome, saturated solution of boric acid, Metaphen, Zephiran,* and *hexylresorcinol solution. Hydrogen peroxide* is also an effective antiseptic but should not be applied to a fresh wound because it may bring about clotting or other undesirable effects.

Sulfa preparations and antibiotics are effective on the skin against microorganisms, but should be used under a doctor's supervision because of possible side effects, including allergic reactions and the danger of making germs resistant to the drugs. *See also* BORIC ACID; MEDICINE CHEST; POISONING; WOUNDS.

► Drugs and Their Uses, *Disinfectants and Antiseptics,* 903; Home Care of Common Ailments, *Local Antiseptics,* 1675; The Skin, *Antiseptics,* 2127.

ANTITOXIN, a substance which counteracts the effect of toxins or poisons in the body produced by harmful organisms, such as bacteria that cause disease. Antitoxins may be developed by the body itself or by the blood of an animal which has been injected with a toxin. Some of the blood is then withdrawn and the serum containing the antitoxin separated from it. This serum or antitoxin may then be injected into a person suffering from the particular infection.

Antitoxins are specific for certain infections. Each bacterial toxin may be counteracted only by the antitoxin effective against it, not by any other which may be potent against other disease-causing toxins.

Diphtheria antitoxin, specific both for curative and preventive purposes, is regarded as one of the greatest of all medical discoveries. Moreover, improved methods are now in general use. One of these

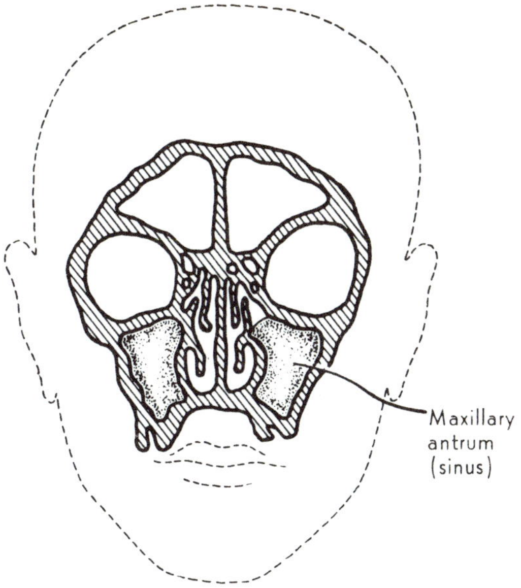

Antrum—The large sinuses at the sides of the nose in the jaws are called *maxillary sinuses.* They are located in a bone known as the *maxilla,* which is the upper jawbone.

consists of injection of *diphtheria toxoid,* a mixture of toxin and antitoxin which causes the body to develop its own antitoxin without actually suffering from the acute disease itself.

Antitoxins are also available against *botulism, scarlet fever, tetanus, staphylococcal infections* and *snakebite.* They have also been effective in *erysipelas, meningitis,* and *epidemic sore throat.* Penicillin and the sulfonamide drugs have provided such powerful chemical remedies against a number of these infections that many antitoxins are no longer used. *See also* IMMUNITY; IMMUNIZATION.

ANTRUM, a cavity or hollow space, usually within a bone. Most frequently it refers to the *maxillary* *sinus,* one of a pair of sinuses, in the upper jaw. Among others are the *mastoid antrum,* the *pyloric* and the *dental antrums. See also* SINUSES.

ANURIA, the suppression of urine by the kidneys, caused by an obstruction in the urinary tract or a lack of renal function.

ANUS, the extremity of the rectum and the outlet of the bowel.

ANXIETY, a state of mental distress, usually unconscious, that may contain feelings of anticipated helplessness, humiliation, guilt, and worthlessness. Anxiety is one of the commonest psychopathological symptoms of a neurosis. Often the mental distress is low in intensity, but it may be almost continuous. The person suffering from anxiety may feel overconcern about practically everything, both important and unimportant. This has been called *free-floating anxiety.* In such a case the person may claim that he cannot think clearly and his concentration is poor. There may be feelings of weakness, perspiration may be profuse, and pupils may enlarge.

Anxiety may be diverted to one or more organs of the body, appearing in the individual in the guise of a physical symptom. When mental distress is turned into a physical manifestation, it is called *conversion hysteria.*

Anxiety may also manifest itself in a specific fear or *phobia*, which is completely out of proportion to the actual danger. Thus, fear of being left alone in a room may represent unconscious anxiety over being abandoned and helpless. Here the unconscious conflict of the mind is related to something specific in the environment. Anxiety dreams are common, often resulting in nightmares. While the dreamer is aware of the content of the dream, the unconscious mental distress is obscured. As in all methods of dealing with anxiety, the person attempts to protect himself from the real causes by withdrawing the conflict from awareness into his subconscious.

Different from the free-floating anxiety described above is the *anxiety attack,* whereby the individual is thrown into a sudden state of intense anxiety which may last a few minutes or less and then subsides. Such attacks are frequently the complaint of mentally disturbed people. During such attacks the patient may be afraid of dying, or of having heart disease or cancer. Often he is in the grip of anxiety without knowing why, only that the "walls are closing in on him," that he is helpless in a gigantic, threatening world. Anxiety attacks are often accompanied by bodily symptoms, such as palpitation, difficulty in breathing, perspiration, coldness of the extremities, headaches, etc.

Treatment of anxiety may involve extensive psychotherapy in severe neurosis. The therapist recognizes that the symptoms are the end product of the patient's mental conflicts, and focuses his attention on the patient's life problems, helping him to reorganize his personality so that as the patient grows stronger, his symptoms will disappear without primary attention.

Children's fears, like adults', fall into two main groups: normal fears of real and immediate dangers and fears—more properly called anxieties—of imaginary dangers. For example, it is quite normal for children to be afraid of hurting themselves by a fall if they find themselves high up in a tree. But if a child is terrified of climbing anything at all and frightened by every little casual tumble, this is no longer normal fear; it is anxiety.

Transitory anxieties are common to most people throughout life. In varying degrees children seem to go through periods when they are afraid of dangers that do not really threaten them, such as the doctor, the policeman, animals, death, being left alone. They may also be frightened by creatures of their own invention. To understand childhood anxieties parents need to know that these menacing fantasy figures and other imaginary threats represent, at least in part, the child's belief that he somehow deserves to be punished. Even though his parents are kind and loving, a four-year-old can't help feeling that it is wrong of him to be so jealous of the baby or to have a strong impulse to do something "bad" of which his parents (and therefore his own conscience) will not approve. As children gradually gain mastery over their anti-

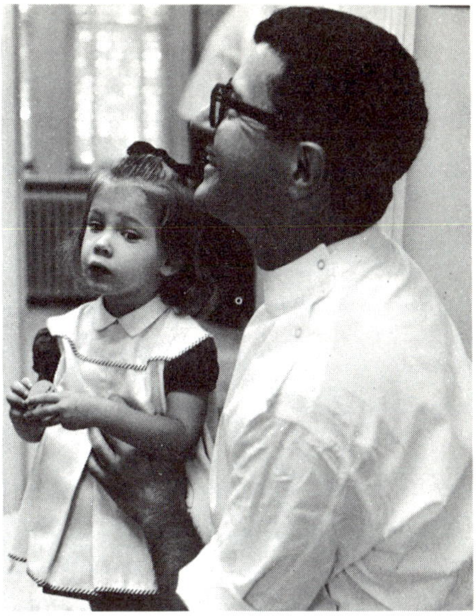

Anxiety in Children — The little girl's fear of the dentist may be a mixture of normal fear of real pain and of anxiety, or fear of imaginary danger. Anxieties will lessen as knowledge of life and reality increases.

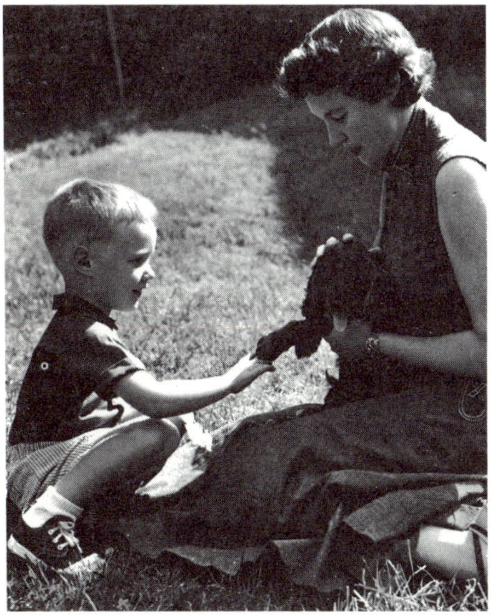

Anxiety in Children — In trying to accustom young children to animals, it is usually best to start with a small animal, such as a kitten, puppy or rabbit.

social impulses and as their sense of reality grows through greater knowledge of life, anxieties tend either to fade or to disappear. *See also* EMOTIONAL HEALTH; FEAR; MENTAL DEPRESSION; STRESS.

► Stress and Disease, *The Relation of Anxiety and Mood Depression to the Primary Emotional States,* 2215.

ANXIETY IN INFANTS. Sometime between six and ten months, many infants suddenly turn shy and begin to act differently to strangers than to the adults they're used to. Babies who had been perfectly friendly and playful with outsiders now either stare distrustfully at an unfamiliar person, bury their heads, or begin to cry. (Other babies, of course, just retain their old outgoing response.) This fear reaction to strangers, what psychologists call "eight-months-anxiety," is often unexpected and upsetting to parents. But it's not a sign that something has gone wrong. On the contrary, it means a new stage in the child's development. The anxiety simply shows that he's now able to distinguish familiar faces from strange ones, and that he strongly prefers those he knows, such as his mother's or father's. It's the first indication of attachment, the beginning of love.

It also indicates that he recognizes the meaning of separation. A baby who formerly didn't seem to mind at all when his mother went out will, during this anxiety period, begin to cry as soon as he sees her getting ready to leave without him. He's not yet developed to the point where he's sure she will return. Playing the simple game of peek-a-boo can help him gain confidence in the feeling that "Mother-goes-away-but-comes-back-again." Another thing that's generally helpful is to have more than one person taking care of the baby. All parents need to get away now and then, and it's easier if the baby has grown accustomed to two or three other people. More than that may confuse him. Though this sudden shyness may be inconvenient or occasionally embarrassing for parents, it should be welcomed as a sign of the child's mental and emotional growth.

ANXIETY IN INFANTS — At some time between six and eight months, a baby often becomes shy, anxious, even fearful in the presence of strangers. This may occur even with infants who have previously been perfectly at ease and outgoing with everyone they have met. By six months, however, the infant has begun to notice facial details and has learned to distinguish the familiar from the strange. He develops a definite preference for the familiar, so that now when a strange face appears, he may express surprise and distrust. This anxiety is perfectly natural, so natural in fact that psychologists have a term for it: "eight-months-anxiety." Parents, especially when they are planning to leave the baby in the care of a baby-sitter, must learn to recognize this period of anxiety and to realize that it may reappear from time to time throughout the early years of his childhood.

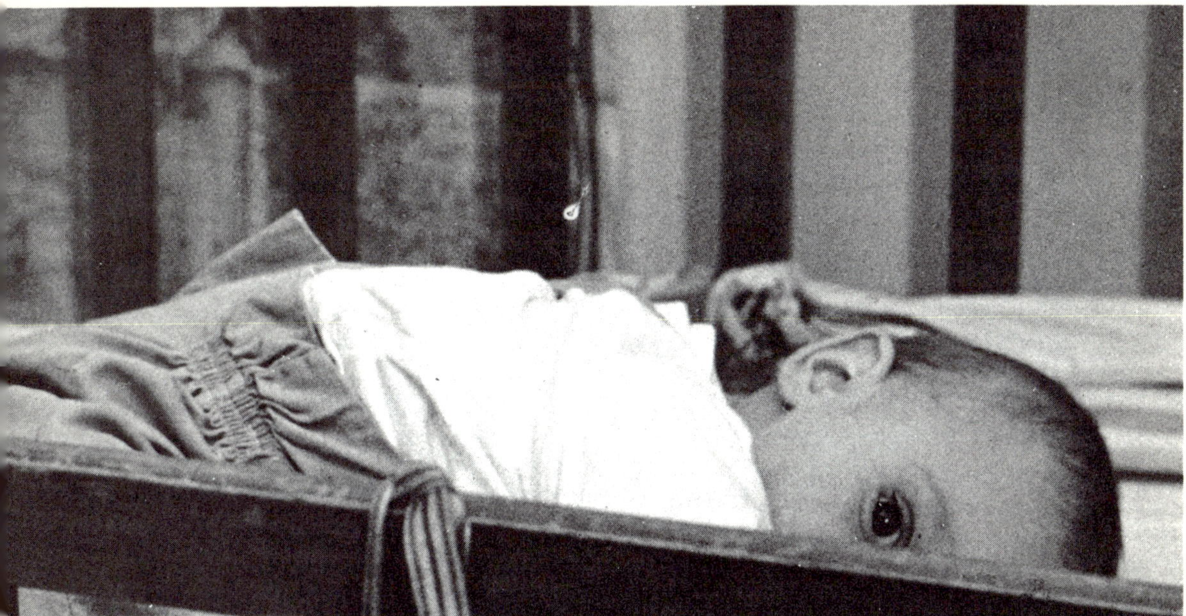

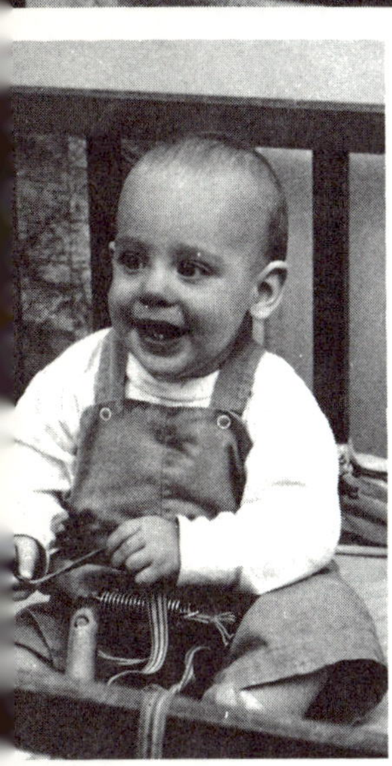

An infant is so competely dependent on his parents for love and comfort and for all his physical needs that any absence on their part may be alarming to him until he comes to learn that they definitely will return. Especially if he is passing through the eight-month anxiety stage, he is apt to resent any face that is not a beloved, familiar one. When a visitor approaches him, the child may look up expecting to see one of his parents and then burst into dismayed tears when he sees that it is someone else.

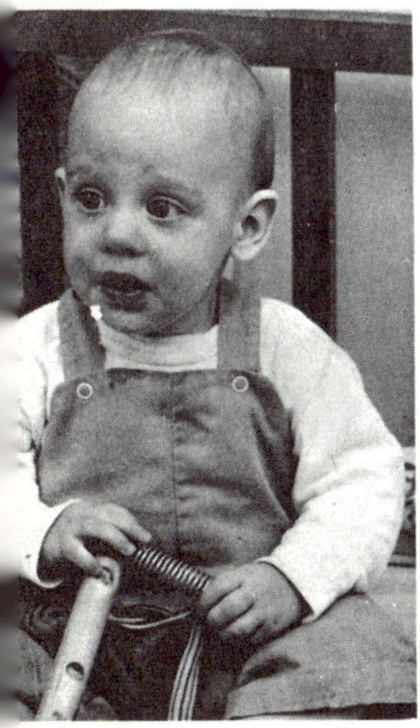

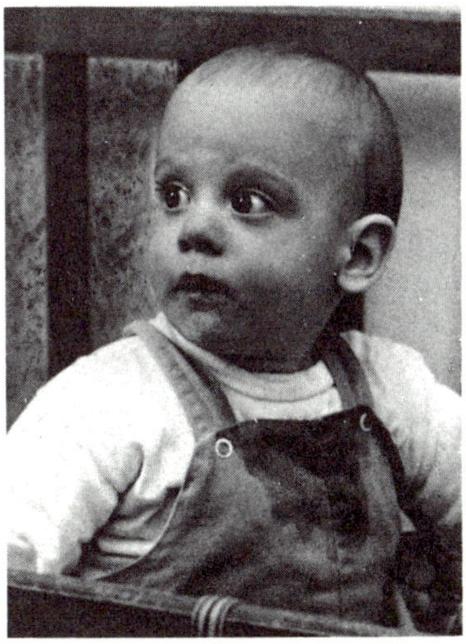

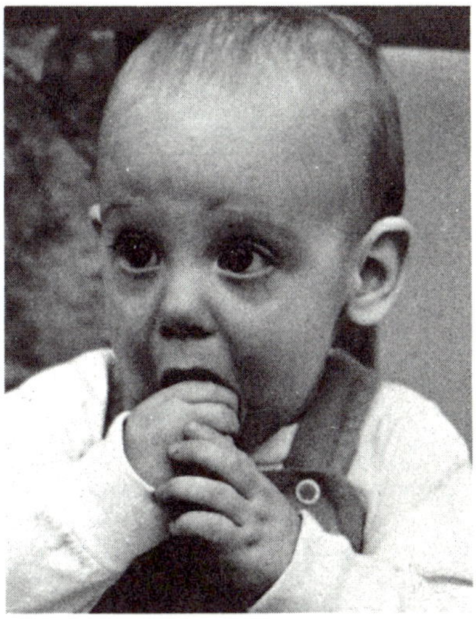

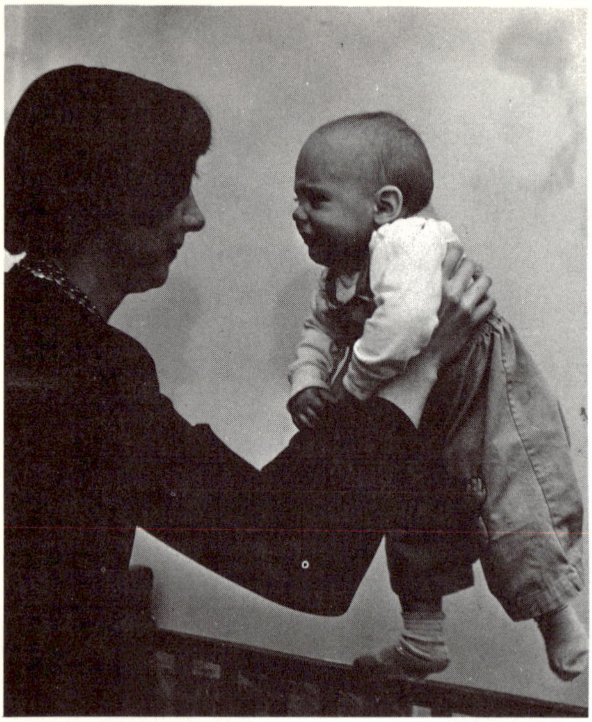

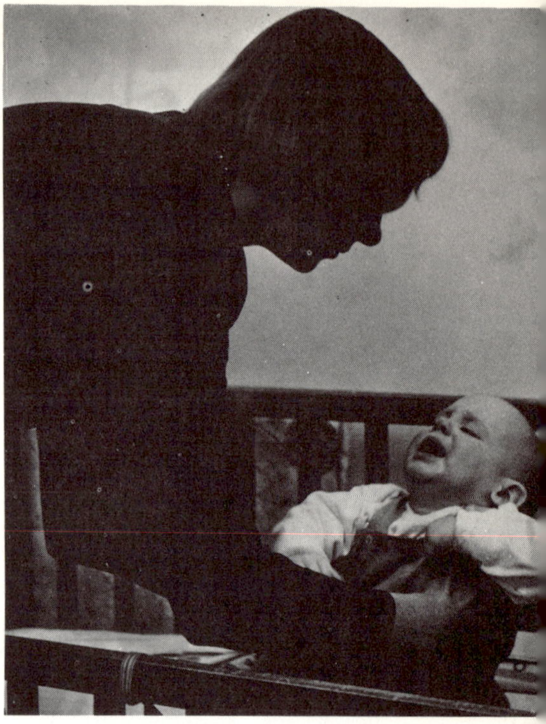

An attempt to pick him up will usually result in more howls, even if the visitor is someone he accepted previously. Coaxing is useless. It is best to leave the child to his own devices while Mother, near him, chats to the visitor. Reassured by his mother's presence, after a little while he may forget his fear as curiosity overcomes it, and he may approach the visitor at his own pace. It is still best to go slowly, because an over-hasty approach may set off the tears again.

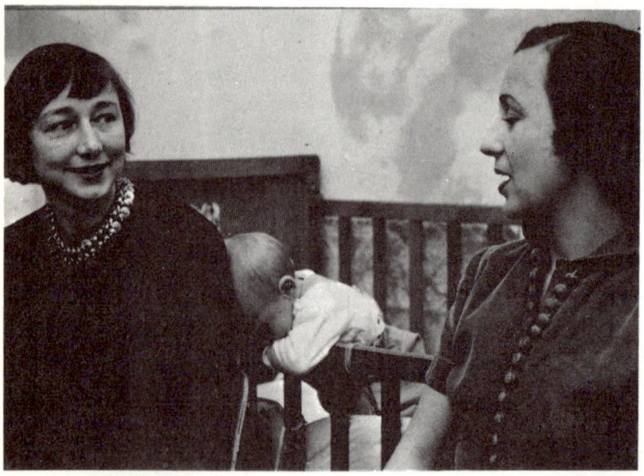

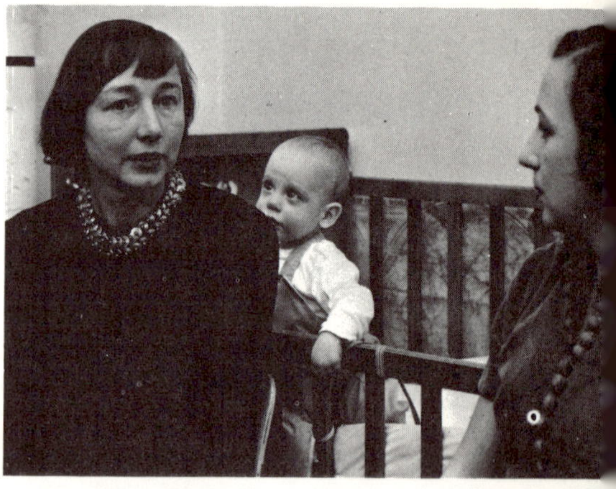

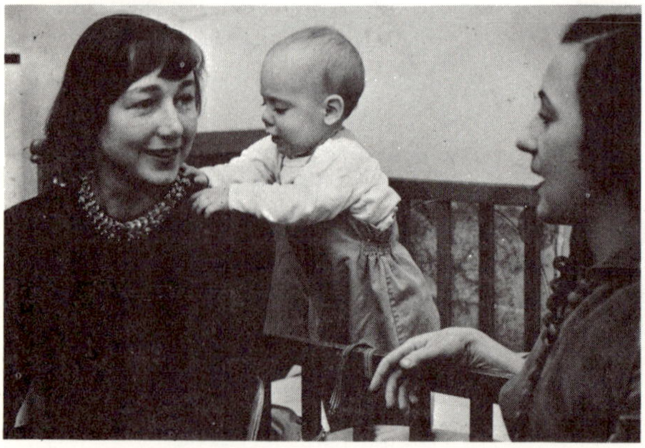

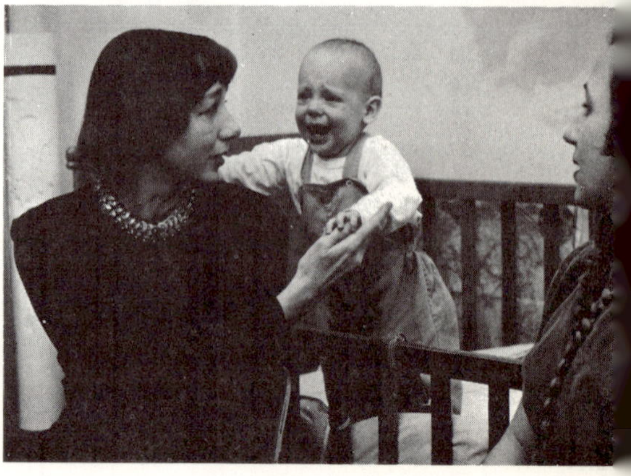

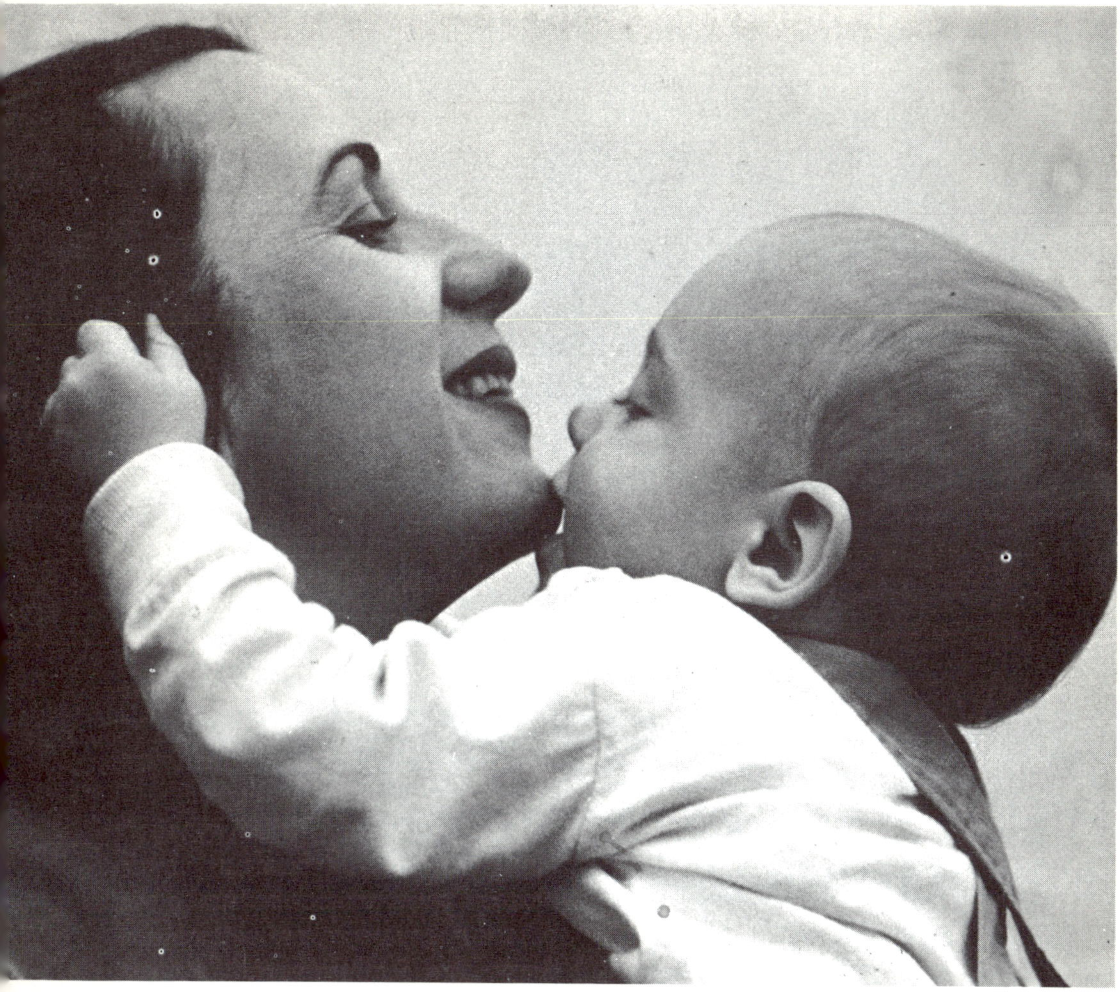

A hug from mother will comfort him; then, seated safely in her lap, his fears forgotten, he will feel the necessary support to overcome his anxiety about the visitor. With no one trying to hurry him he will be able to relax and enjoy his natural curiosity and eager desire for new experiences. Eight-month anxiety, although it may upset and sometimes embarrass parents, is not a serious matter. It is a sign of the child's new awareness of the distinction between familiar and strange faces and the meaning of separation. It is the first indication of attachment and love.

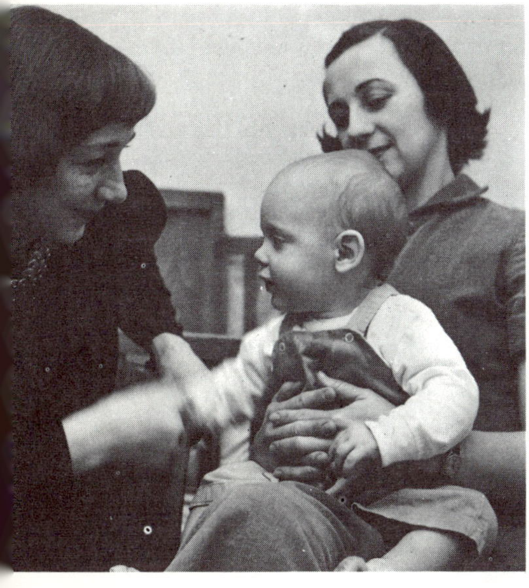

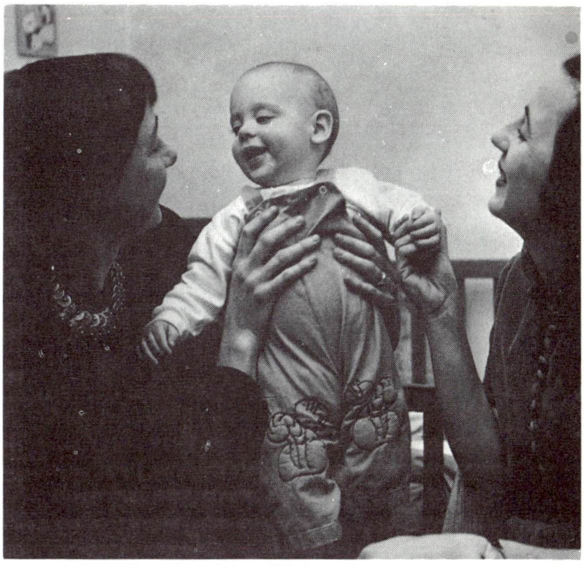

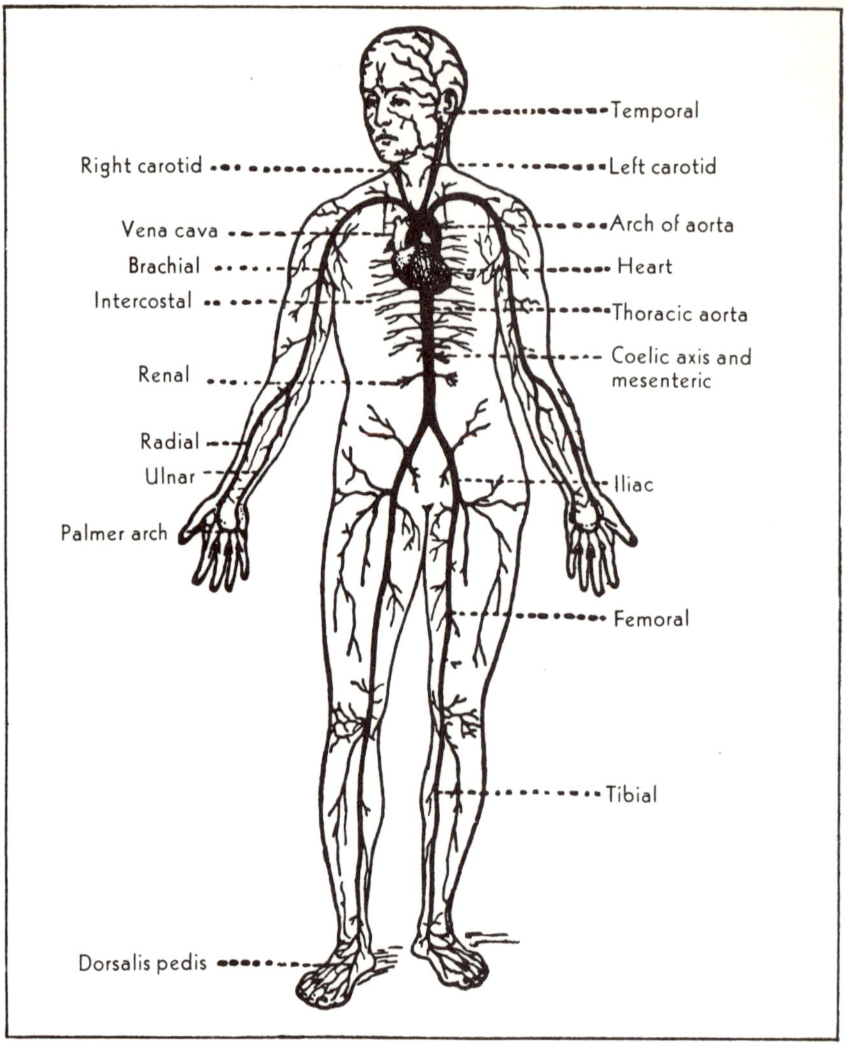

Aorta—The aorta is the largest artery of the body. As it projects up out of the heart, it makes an arch to the left and courses downward behind the heart to the abdomen where it branches off into two vessels, one extending down each leg. The arch is called the *arch of the aorta*. Large vessels branch off the arch and go to the head, neck, and down the arms. The aorta carries oxygenated blood from the heart to all parts of the body.

AORTA, the largest blood vessel coming from the heart. It distributes blood to every part of the body through its system of arteries. *See also* CIRCULATORY SYSTEM.

APC VIRUSES. During the summer of 1955 outbreaks occurred in several American communities and later in England of a condition in which there was sore throat, moderate fever and intense reddening of the eyes. A new group of viruses was isolated known as *APC viruses* or *adenoidal, pharyngial* and *conjunctival viruses.* Infections with these organisms which may occur as epidemics have been found in outbreaks in sore throats and red eyes in children and also with atypical pneumonia in soldiers. The condition usually clears up without any fatality. *See also* VIRUSES.

APHASIA, an organic condition caused by lesions in the cortex of the brain which produces loss or impairment of the capacity to use words as symbols of ideas. *See also* ALEXIA; APHONIA.

APHONIA, loss of voice because of hysteria or peripheral lesion. *See also* APHASIA.

APHRODISIAC, any preparation or agent which allegedly stimulates sexual desire. Actually desire is mostly mental so that drugs which release inhibitions may act as aphrodisiacs. Certain substances which have an irritating effect when excreted may stimulate congestion of the sex organs. *See also* CANTHARIDES.

APLASTIC ANEMIA. *See* RED BLOOD CELLS, DISEASES OF.

APOCRINE GLANDS. *See* SKIN; BODY ODOR.

APOPLEXY. In apoplexy, or "stroke" or cerebral hemorrhage, an artery in the brain either ruptures and bleeds or is blocked. The victim is apt to lose consciousness and some part of the body is paralyzed, at least temporarily. Apoplexy occurs most frequently in persons whose arteries have deteriorated with age or who have high blood pressure. Age tends to bring rising blood pressure and degenerative change in the arteries. As the proportion of elderly people in the United States increases, the proportion of people susceptible to apoplexy also increases and therefore apoplexy has become a leading cause of death. When younger persons have apoplexy it is frequently the result of a blood clot from elsewhere in the body obstructing a blood vessel which serves the brain. This obstruction has the same effect as an actual hemorrhage of blocking the flow of blood in the brain.

Apoplexy occurs in various ways. Especially with older persons, apoplexy may take place during a regular nightly sleep, with no apparent external cause. Sometimes apoplexy is associated with an emotional outburst, a sudden intense effort or acute stress. Without warning, a person may collapse suddenly. Partial paralysis is a typical consequence, regardless of the way apoplexy occurs.

Emergency assistance to a victim of apoplexy begins by putting him to bed immediately. He should lie supine and if he is unconscious be placed on his side. If he is placed on his back during unconsciousness, his tongue may fall back into his throat, interfere with breathing, and cause strangulation. A doctor should be summoned promptly.

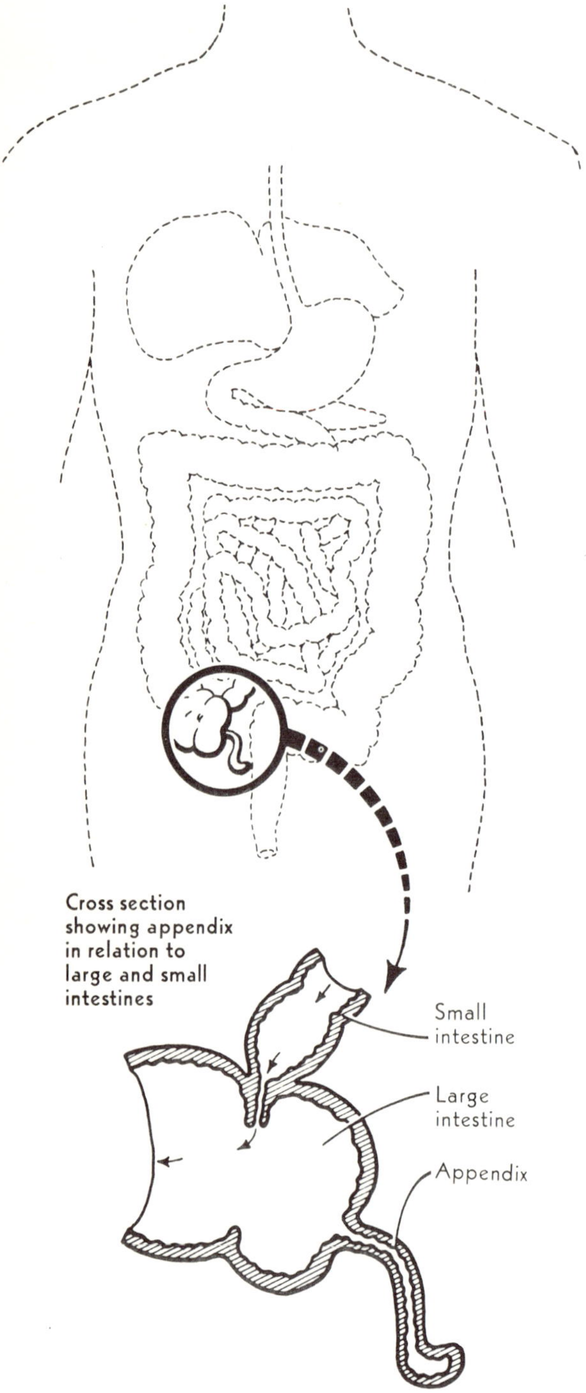

Appendicitis—The appendix is a small sac attached to the colon which causes trouble out of all proportion to its size.

As long as the stricken person is unconscious, fluids and foods must be given artifically; liquids will have to be injected and food injected through tubes into the veins. These measures and others are prescribed and administered by the doctor.

The extent of paralysis can be established only after the person has regained consciousness, and sometimes a long period of time must elapse before the full extent of the paralysis is determined. Paralysis due to a temporary condition, such as pressure on a nerve, rather than to actual destruction of nerve tissue will disappear with recovery. The body, if adequate care is provided, tends to mend such damage and to restore power of movement lost for temporary reasons. A person crippled by apoplexy can be rehabilitated in most instances if the proper treatment is begun at the right time. The patient should always be handled very carefully and gently, never abruptly pushed or jerked into position. His position must be changed every few hours in order to prevent the formation of bed sores and ulcers and the skin should be kept perfectly clean at all times, including a complete bath each day. *See also* CHOREA; EMBOLISM; PARALYSIS; THROMBOSIS; CIRCULATORY SYSTEM; ARTERIOSCLEROSIS. *See* MEDIGRAPH page 2233.

APPENDICITIS, inflammation of the appendix, more properly known as the *vermiform appendix*, a finger-shaped sac three to six inches long

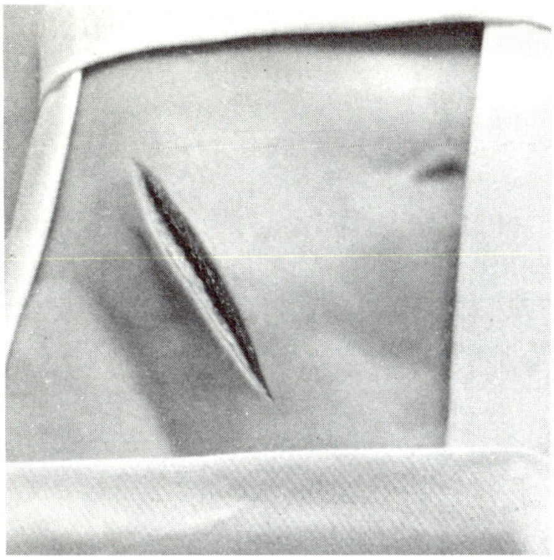

Incision—After the skin has been disinfected, an incision is made down to the muscle. The incision is on the right side a few inches from the groin.

which projects from the large bowel, in the lower right quarter of the abdomen.

Infection and inflammation of the appendix are potentially serious because the infection may spread to the *peritoneum,* the membranous tissue which lines the abdomen. Acute *peritonitis,* or inflammation of the peritoneum, is a grave development and may be fatal unless treated promptly.

Peritonitis may result from appendicitis in at least two ways. The peritoneum is shaped to fit over the appendix, just as a glove covers a finger, and is thus in close contact with it. Accordingly infection of the appendix may spread to the peritoneum simply by contact. Moreover, if an inflamed appendix is left untreated, it may rupture or develop *gangrene.* In either case, masses of infected matter will be discharged into the peritoneal cavity.

APPENDICITIS

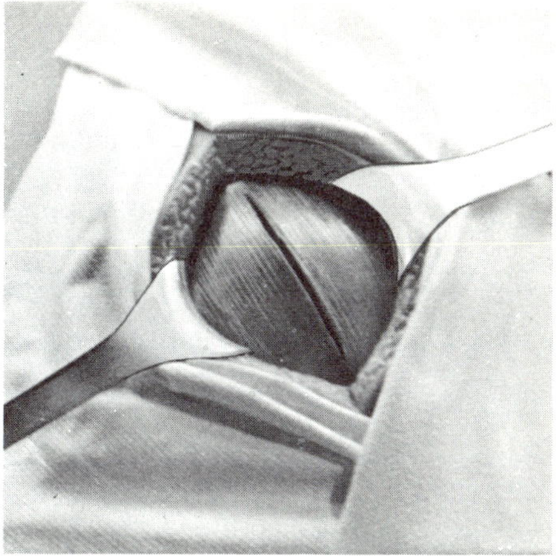

Surgical Field—Sterile towels are brought to the edges of the incision so that only the surgical field is exposed. This minimizes the danger of contamination. After the skin and fat are pulled back by retractors, the first layer of muscle is exposed. The muscle is cut in the direction of its fibers.

These possibilities demand that the condition be accorded immediate attention by a physician. Delay often unnecessarily permits the development of complications, renders treat-

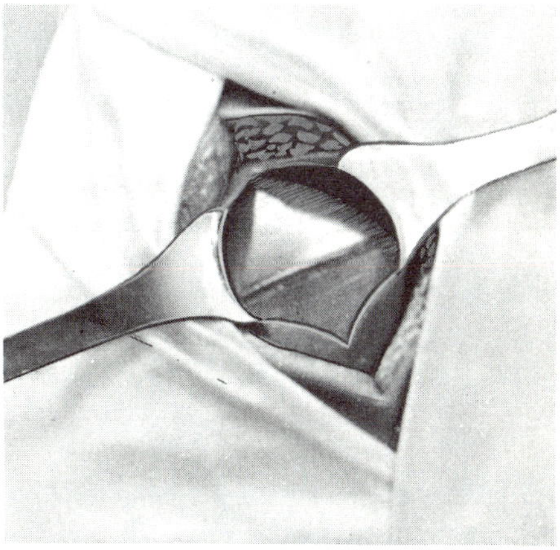

Retracting Muscle—The outer layer of muscle is also retracted, bringing the second layer into view. The fibers of the second layer run in a different direction than those of the first layer. Again a cut is made along the grain of the muscle.

the disease and its causes Appendicitis is an inflammatory disease of the appendix. It can occur at any age but appears most often in young adults of both sexes.

The exact cause is unknown, but one of the explanations offered is the bacterial cause, that is, bacterial infection elsewhere in the body may be carried by the blood or by food to the appendix. A more acceptable theory is based on a mechanical cause, in which the appendix is blocked, usually by stool or, rarely, by swallowed foreign bodies.

Occasionally worms may lodge in the appendix and cause infection.

In all cases the symptoms are the same: the appendix is infected and swollen, and acts like an abscess on any part of the body.

symptoms The accompanying Medi-Graph diagrams one specific appendicitis attack. However, it must be emphasized that there is *no* typical case of acute appendicitis. The appendix may be in an unusual location and the area of pain may be completely different from that described. Occasionally the pain is located on the left side of the abdomen. For very old people appendicitis may be almost painless. Since it is difficult to make a diagnosis, no increasing abdominal pain should be disregarded.

complications The common complication is rupture of the appendix. When this happens the infection can spread to the membrane lining of the abdomen. The resulting peritonitis can severely infect the whole abdominal area. Before the rupture there is a great increase in pain and a spread of the area of pain.

Another complication is that the appendix may perforate and an abscess form in the area of the infection. This may burst into other organs or even open through the skin surface in the form of a fistula.

Abscess of the liver and abscess below the right diaphragm also are possible complications.

prevention (or lessening of impact) There is no way to prevent appendicitis. Once the attack begins, prompt medical care and surgery are essential in order to avoid serious complications and speed recovery. The patient should avoid taking any laxatives, because they can cause the infected appendix to rupture. Ice packs may ease the pain, and even slow the process, but surgery is the only cure. So-called chronic appendicitis, in which there are repeated attacks, is very unusual, and most physicians do not believe such a condition exists.

Appendicitis and Peritonitis

1. Appendicitis . . .

A. In typical cases, starts with off-and-on pain near navel.

B. Pain radiates down to right lower abdomen over appendix. Becomes constant and progressively more severe. Spot is tender to touch.

C. Nausea and occasionally vomiting follows. Sequence may take anywhere from several hours to 1-2 days.

D. Blood test reveals inflammation.

E. Attack may pass by itself. But if it gets worse . . .

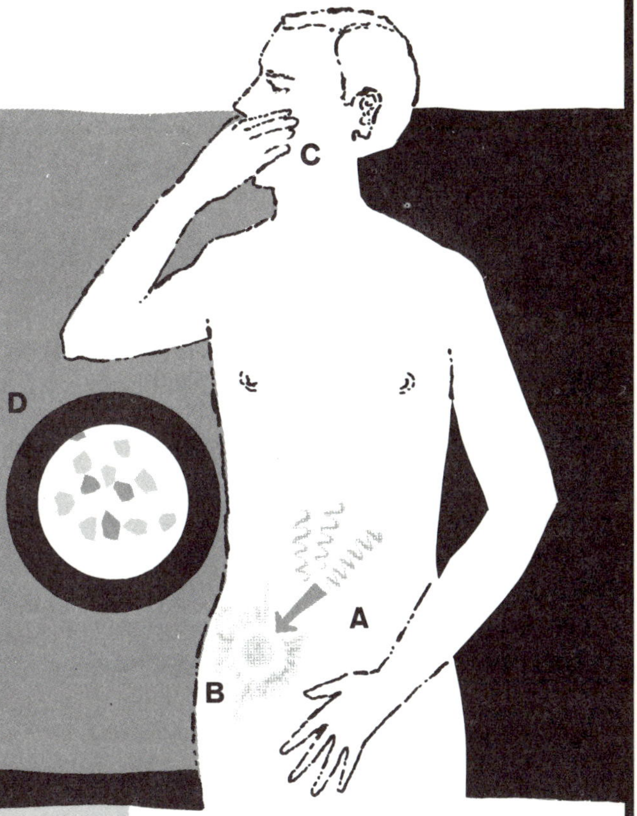

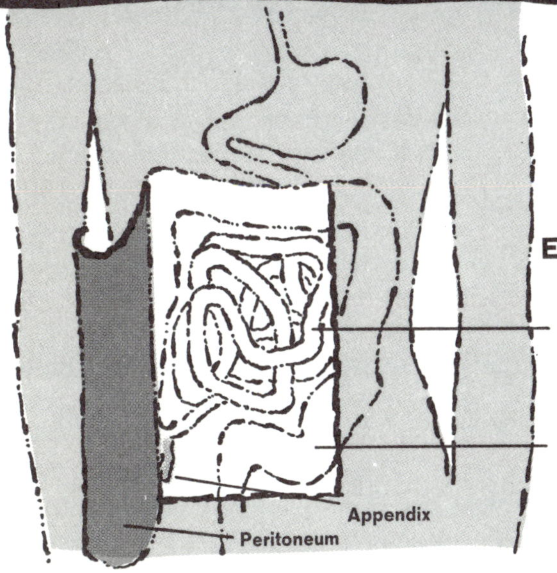

2. . . . and Peritonitis

. . . infection from badly inflamed or bursting appendix may spread to peritoneum (membrane lining of abdomen). Resulting peritonitis may severely infect whole abdominal area.

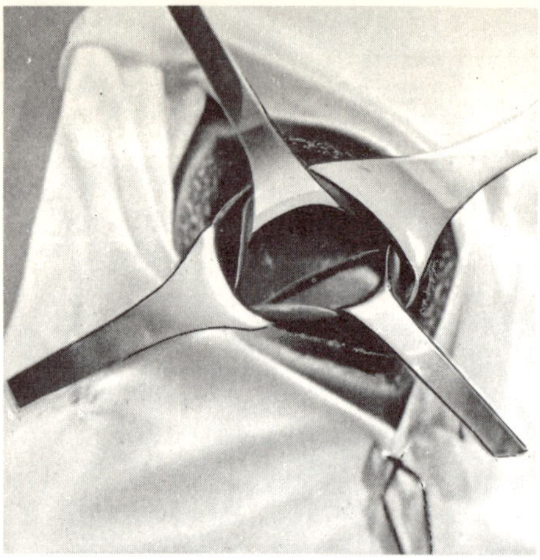

Peritoneum—When the second muscle layer is retracted, a glistening membrane, the *peritoneum,* is exposed. The peritoneum lines the abdominal cavity.

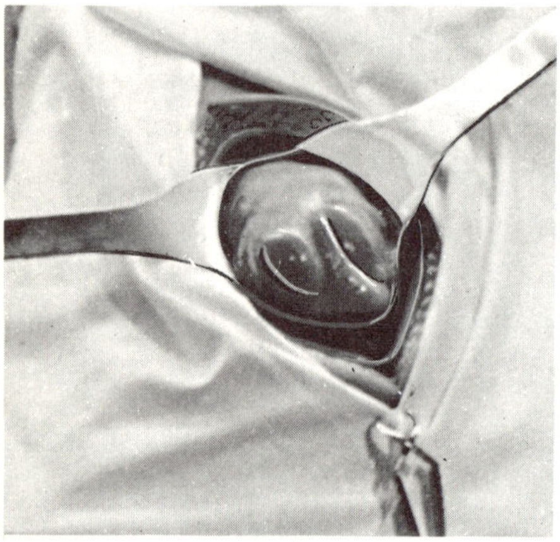

Cecum—The peritoneum has been cut and the first part of the colon is brought into the wound. This part of the colon is called the *cecum.*

Appendix—Attached to the cecum is the *appendix.* Its blood supply is cut off and it is about to be cut away between two clamps. Clamps are used to prevent contents from spilling out.

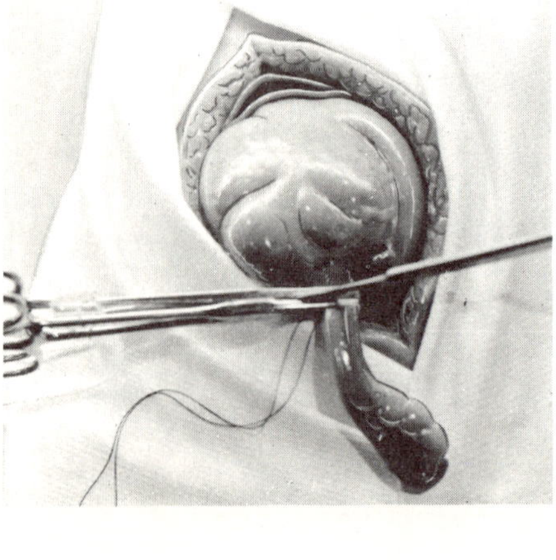

ment more difficult, and may possibly endanger life. Attempts to diagnose and treat the symptoms of appendicitis without a physician, by ascribing the symptoms to a gastrointestinal disturbance and administering a cathartic or laxative, may have serious consequences. Abdominal pain should never be treated with a cathartic or laxative without the cause of the pain being first established.

Appendicitis usually begins with a sick feeling, accompanied by nausea, lack of appetite, and at first a rather diffuse abdominal soreness. Vomiting may occur, and a rise in temperature is likely. Gradually the pain tends to concentrate on the right side of the abdomen below the navel and the muscles in that region tighten when pressed in examination.

Symptoms indicative of appendicitis can actually arise from nothing more serious than accumulation of gas or solid matter in a part of the bowel. However, ordinarily these symptoms disappear with elimination from the bowel. If they persist, the doctor should be promptly consulted. He will determine whether or not appendicitis has actually occurred. Examination of the blood will usually show abnormal numbers of white cells if the appendix is infected.

Diagnosis is not always easy because of the variety of difficulties which may manifest similar symptoms. This is especially true of the resemblance between the early stages of appendicitis and, in some cases, of early *pneumonia.* In early pneumonia, inflammation in the lower lungs may spread to the *diaphragm,* the large breathing muscle which walls off the chest and abdominal cavities from each other. Pain is present in the same part of the abdomen as in appendicitis, and is also accompanied by rigidity on touch.

Because of the danger presented by an inflamed appendix, surgery is a common and satisfactory means of eliminating the condition. Appendectomy is so completely standardized that recovery will usually be normal, if the operation takes place before the appendix ruptures.

If the appendix has ruptured, or has become gangrenous, however, the situation is much more serious. Ordinarily, in a simple appendectomy, the patient will be up in two or three days, and sent home from the hospital in a week. When complications occur, the condition demands different considerations and may involve much more time. Fortunately the antibiotic drugs such as *penicillin, terramycin, aureomycin,* and others control peritonitis so that death from this complication is now rare.

The precise way in which appendicitis develops is not fully understood. Doctors once believed that it was the result of food lodging in the appendix. Many appendices removed and examined were found to contain a variety of unexpected objects and materials, such as stones, hair, seeds, pins, bones, lead

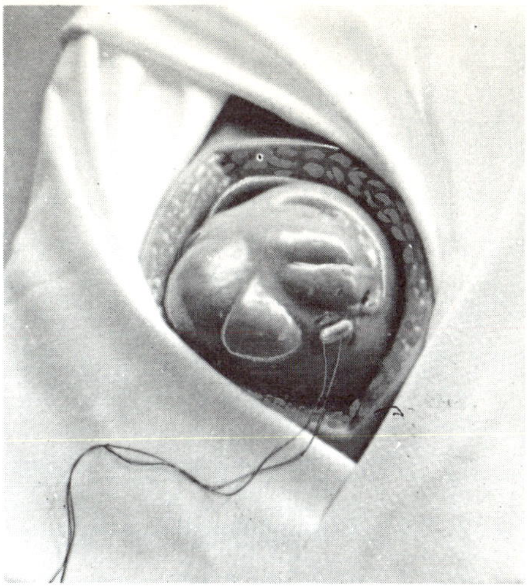

Sutures—The ends of the stumps are turned in and the purse string sutures are drawn taut and tied.

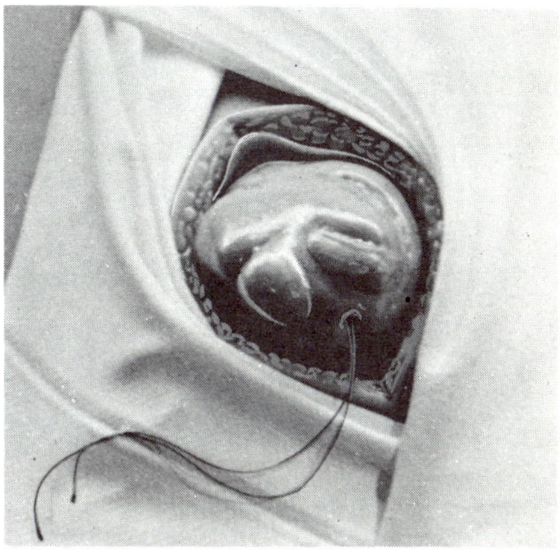

Stump of Appendix—A dimple shows where the stump of the appendix has been inverted. The smooth surface remaining prevents the cecum from adhering to the peritoneum.

Closing the Peritoneum—After the neighboring parts of the intestine are examined for perforations, the bowel is put back in the abdomen and the peritoneum closed.

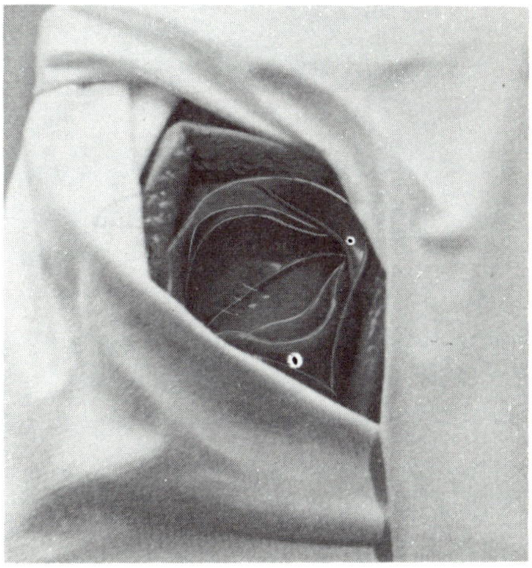

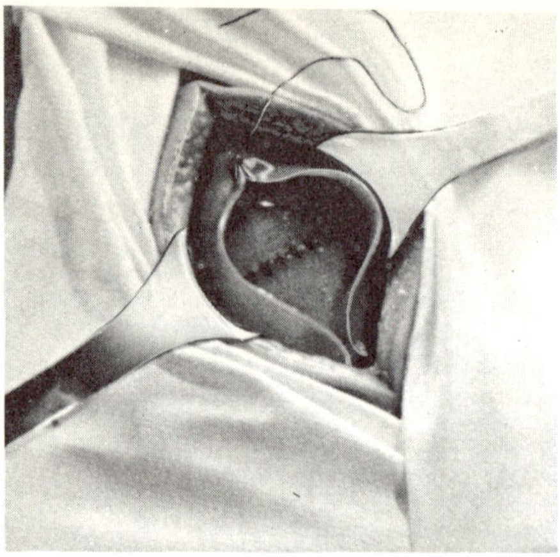

Sutures—The cut surfaces of each layer are brought together and sutured.

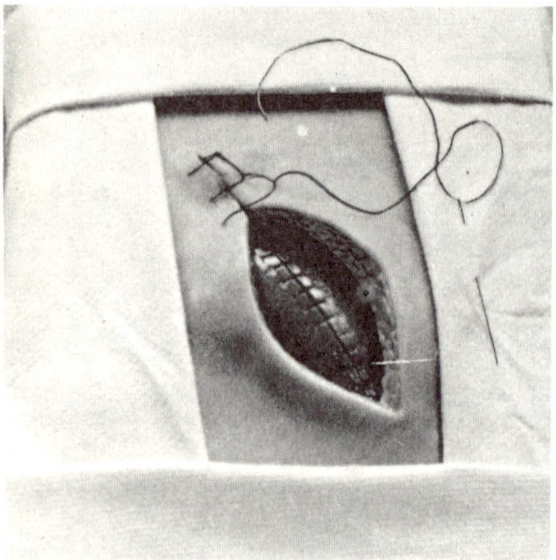

Closing the Wound—The outer part of the wound is about to be closed. Various types of sutures can be used. This one is called *the glover's stitch*.

The Closed Wound—The appearance of the closed wound. With the skin edges placed together, the scar will be minimal.

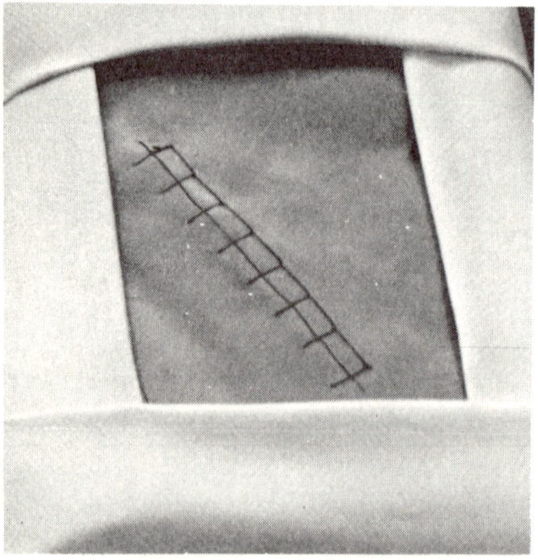

shot, and sometimes worms. Many other appendices, however, did not contain anything foreign. It is now felt that inflammation and infection are commonly caused by germs.

The structure of the appendix, with its long slender tube, narrow opening at one end only, and lining of lymphatic tissue, makes it susceptible to inflammatory swelling and the resulting closure. The organ then cannot empty its contents. An abscess forms, the swelling increases, and the accumulating infected and lymphatic matter within the tube

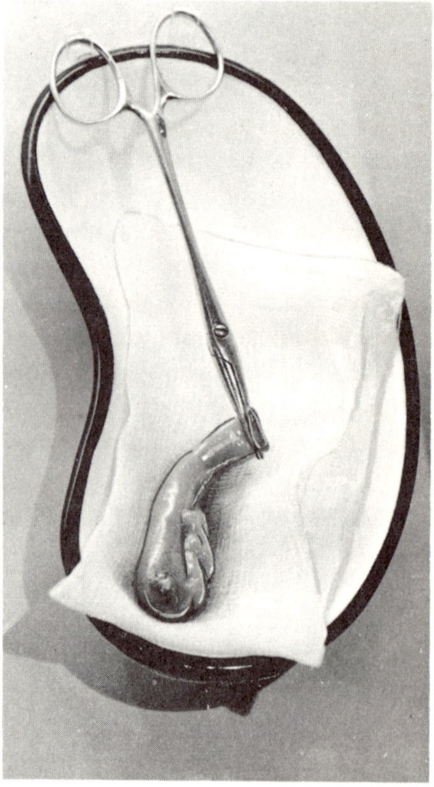

Pathology—The appendix will be sent to the laboratory to be examined by the pathologist. The appendix measures about three inches long.

cannot escape. The appendix may then burst or become gangrenous. Gangrene is the atrophy of the tissues locally affected.

Sudden relief after a period of pain should be considered a potential danger signal rather than a sign of improvement, for it may signify that perforation has occurred or that gangrene has begun.

Appendicitis is a significant threat to health in the United States. It ranks fifteenth among causes of death, and kills sixteen thousand persons annually. If children below the age of fifteen are eliminated from these statistics, appendicitis becomes the eighth or ninth cause of death. *See also* PERITONITIS. *See* MEDIGRAPH page 217.

► Digestion and Digestive Diseases, *Appendicitis,* 863.

APPETITE, the recurring and usually natural desire for food. A distinction must be made between appetite and hunger. Hunger pangs result from contractions of an empty stomach and are rarely felt by anyone who regularly eats adequate amounts of food. Appetite arises with the customary intervals of eating and may be influenced by numerous external and internal phenomena. Eating is one of the most firmly fixed of all habits, and appetite is usually a longing for something one wants to eat at a time when one habitually has or expects food. Ordinarily a good appetite is considered a sign of health.

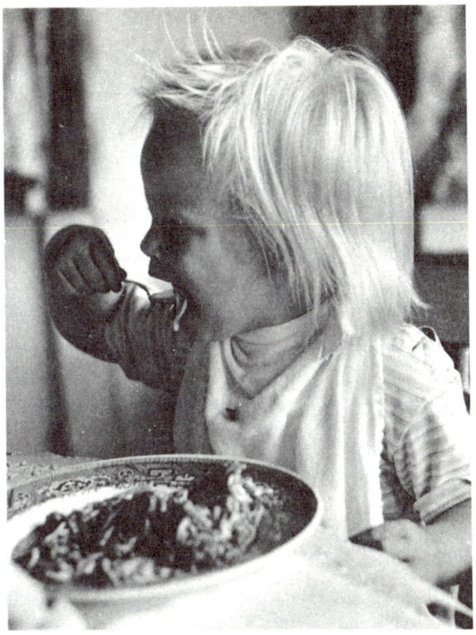

Appetite — Children's bodily needs differ, and often, by his own choice, a child can select the food he requires. A balanced diet is needed, but each meal need not be balanced.

Appetite, however, can become excessive or subject to distorted impulses. Occasionally people suffering from specific disorders, such as diabetes, gastric ulcers, or chronic gastritis, develop appetites out of proportion to their needs. In pregnancy or hysteria, unusual and specialized cravings may develop for particular kinds of foods, or even for injurious substances.

A close connection may exist between appetite and individual psychological experience. Children, for example, are apt to develop cravings without realizing the cause. Eating may be a form of compensation for a major loss or disappointment; or a means of securing attention from adults who otherwise might not notice the child. Some children develop unaccustomed appetite from signifi-

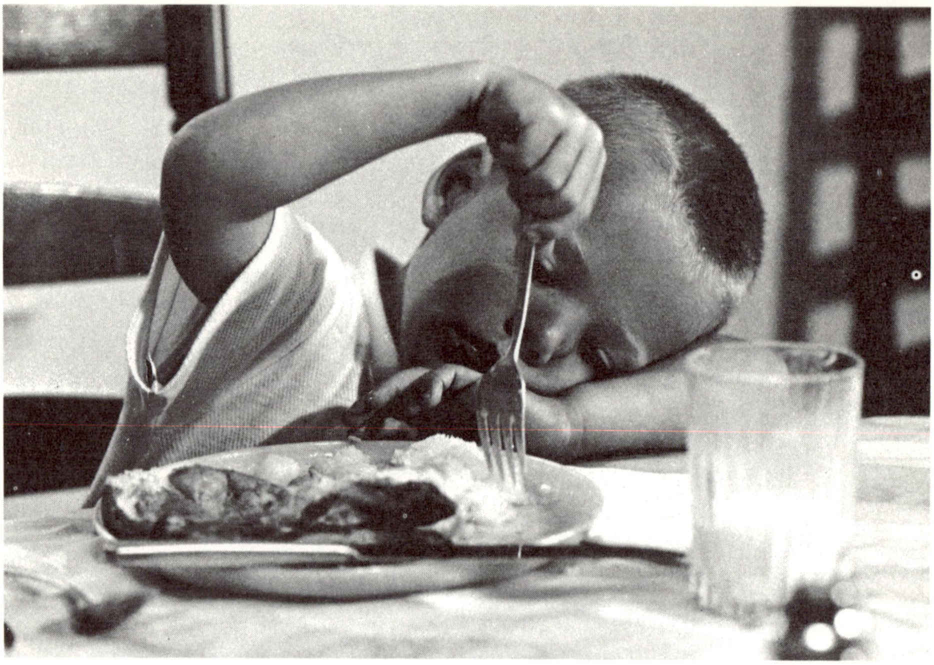

Appetite — A child's appetite will be affected by his rate of growth and activity, by physical and chemical bodily conditions, by moods or feelings, or by fatigue. However, if a child persistently eats too much or too little, parents should consult a doctor.

cant new events taking place about them, such as the birth of a new baby.

A person who has duodenal ulcer seems to have a special form of appetite. His pain is apt to rise and fall with the stomach's desire for food. In such cases, eating tends to relieve the pain, at least temporarily.

Diminution or loss of appetite accompanies many disordered conditions, and is usually one of the symptoms of tuberculosis and anemia. Loss of appetite and refusal to eat anything is known medically as *anorexia nervosa.* Ordinarily this disease is related to some form of emotional instability and is observed more often in women than in men.

Appetite can be artificially decreased by taking such drugs as *Benzedrine* and *Dexedrine.* These drugs are sometimes prescribed for weight reduction, but should be taken only on the advice of a doctor.

Investigation indicates that small amounts of cocktails and other alcoholic drinks arouse or increase appetite, although they hinder the stomach contractions associated with hunger. *See also* ANOREXIA.

APPROVAL. Everyone likes to feel approved of, to have his individuality and his efforts respected. From infancy to adolescence, approval—part of affection—is to a child's personality growth what vitamins—part of good diet—are to his physical growth. While it is comparatively simple to offer a child a balanced diet, however, adults can usually furnish approval only to the degree that they take time to have contact with the child's world.

Adults in a constant rush, for instance, have little time to see in a juvenile artist's fingerpainting anything more than blobs and splashes of color. "How nice," they may say absentmindedly. At the other extreme, a mother who knows her little son's eyes are asking for approval may go into ecstasies over his every creation. The child doesn't feel this as genuine, and praise so easily had can become worthless. How much more meaningful is the tone of voice of the mother or father who has the time to see the creative freedom, the developing awareness of color, and—on the child's own level—the work that has gone into the painting. The tone of a "That's a fine painting, darling," and perhaps the place given on the bulletin board for especially wonderful work constitutes sincere recognition to their youngster.

In its deepest sense, however, approval is not praise for achievement. It is a matter of overall tone and attitude in day-by-day living with children. A youngster takes his first picture of himself from his mother and father, seeing himself as they see him. It is from them he gets his sense of personal worth. This feeling of importance comes more from their basic respect for his intentions and efforts than from admiration for accomplishment. The little girl who glowingly presents her self-tied shoelaces for the first time certainly deserves an admiring "Look at what you've done!" But if the efforts have ended in frustration, she also merits something like "Well, you tried, dear —it takes time to learn."

As a child takes alternately the wobbly steps and giant strides leading to adulthood, real approval lies in showing interest in what he thinks, attention to what he has to say. When he speeds home from school bursting with ideas about democracy, for instance, his concepts may naturally be immature to older people. But for his own phase of growth they can reveal a striking amount of meditation and perception—and they are certainly worthy of responsive discussion. Discussion

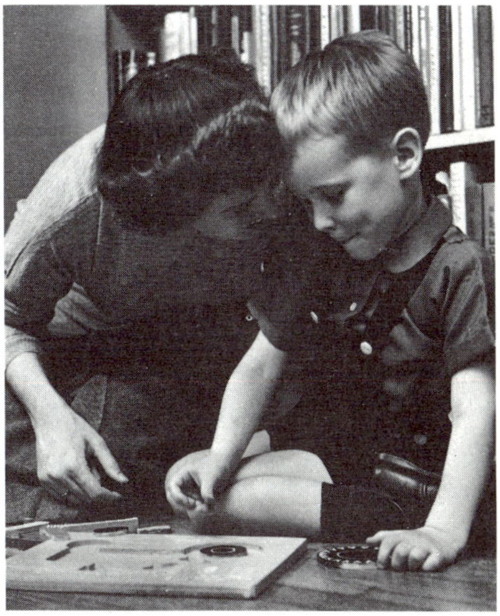

Approval — Approval, an integral part of affection, is essential to a child's personality growth and to his sense of personal worth. Sincere recognition of real achievement or of effort, even when failure results, is of more value than indiscriminate praise.

in itself, even when parents disapprove of some specific ideas, constitutes approval of the way he is growing. Sometimes approval lies in an even simpler act of recognition. When the teen-age girl voluntarily turns to and helps with serving or cleaning up at a party that was purely her parents', just "Thank you" can be applause to her. Her efforts have been recognized and appreciated—not taken for granted.

On the other side of the coin, disapproval must be understood if approval is to be really valuable. For example, some disciplinary measure that is not comprehended by a child is likely to be taken as disapproval of himself personally. A young child in particular should be helped to understand what it is that his parents disapprove of—the act at the time, and not the child himself.

Adults sometimes fear that too much approval will bring about conceit. There is little chance of this. Outward conceitedness arises more from an inner feeling of being personally unimportant. Although all children have their moments of boasting, the youngster who is not sure he is worth while for himself alone is much more likely to brag about how many toys he has than one who has always felt valuable as an individual human being.

The infant, as we know, is concerned with himself. As he grows his concern extends to others. But as a healthy adult he values himself on the same level as other people. A childhood during which he has generally felt approval contributes largely to this balanced attitude.

AQUEOUS HUMOR, the fluid in the front chamber of the eye, between the cornea and the lens. The transparent substance is almost totally water.

ARACHNODACTYLY, derived from the Greek words for spider and finger, a condition in which the fingers and sometimes the toes are abnormally long and thin. This abnormality has a hereditary tendency.

ARGYROL, a proprietary antiseptic drug which contains about 20 per cent silver and proteins found in egg yolk. It is used to control and counteract inflammations of membranes that are secreting or contain mucus.

ARCHES, FALLEN, are due to a breakdown of the natural arch of the foot which is an elastic spring that supports the weight of the entire body. This arch, made up of numerous bones held in place by a series of ligaments and muscles, is a curved structure resembling an arc. Flat feet, a common complaint, may be caused by the natural weakness of the arch, but usually result from certain occupations, injury, or obesity. The condition may be corrected or benefited by wearing proper shoes or arch supports, or by exercises to strengthen the muscles.

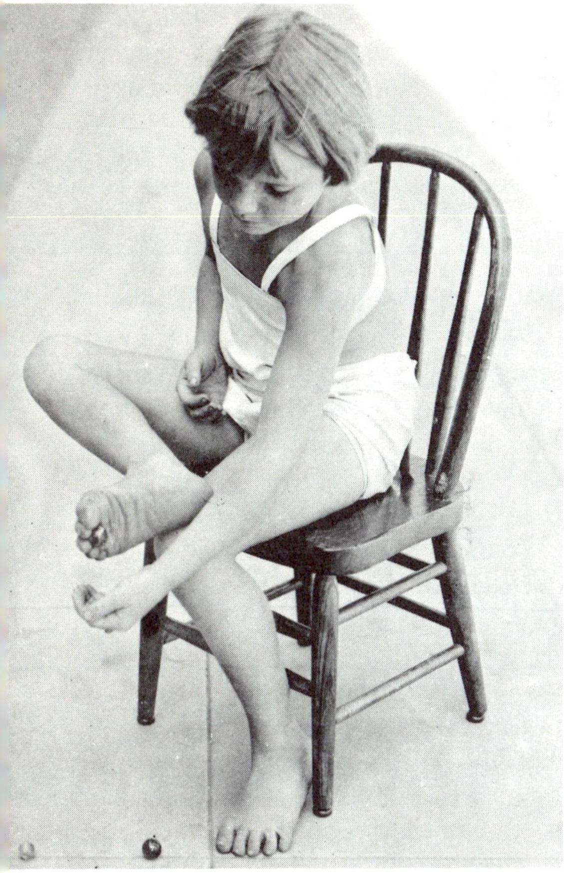

Fallen Arches — An infirmity of the bony arches of the feet results in flat feet. The arch is sunken so that the entire sole is in contact with the ground. The condition of flat feet in a growing child can be corrected by arch supports in shoes and strengthening of the muscles by special exercises. A good corrective exercise for flat feet is being performed by this young girl. The marbles are picked up with the foot and placed in the opposite hand.

ARCTIC HEALTH. The development of aviation greatly increased travel into Arctic regions. Emergency landings may cause people to be exposed without preparation to the unusual climate. These hints may be most helpful in saving life.

The peculiar hazards of the Arctic area relate primarily to cold and snow. Snow blindness is the result of the effects of glare on the eyes. Special goggles are supplied to keep off the glare. The Eskimo makes a snow shield from a scrap of wood; he takes a rectangular piece of thin wood, about six inches long and one inch wide, and burns holes or slits through it at about the width of the eyes. This shield can be placed across the bridge of the nose and held by a piece of string passing around over the ears and in back of the head. Vision is possible through the slits, which serve at the same time to bar the glare of the sun.

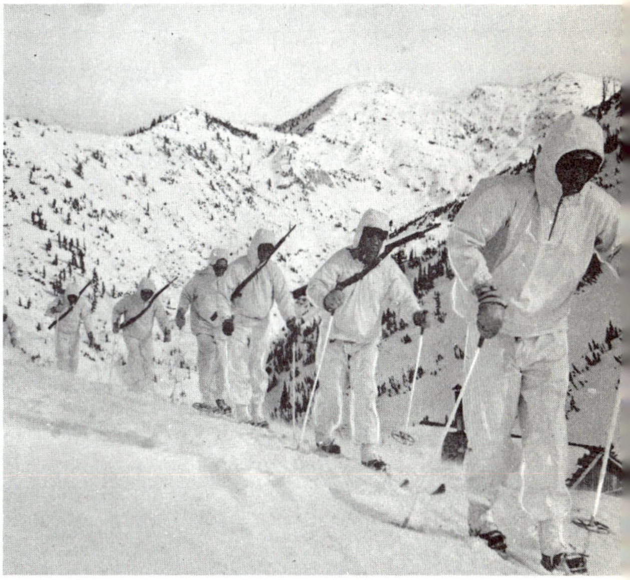

Arctic Health—The human body is able to adapt itself to ordinary changes in temperature. But for extreme temperatures and weather conditions, the body must be protected. These para-ski troopers are dressed properly for the climatic conditions. Because they are surrounded by snow, it is also necessary that they protect their eyes from the reflected glare of the sun. The glare is prevented by their Polaroid goggles.

Another help is the blackening of cheeks and the bridge of the nose with soot, charcoal, or dirty engine oil. This blackening helps to cut down reflections from the sun.

Tight shoes encourage freezing and damage to the feet. The shoes worn in the Arctic regions must be big enough to allow the person to wear at least two pairs of heavy socks. If the shoes are not sufficiently large for this purpose, it is well to remove the shoes entirely and to wrap the feet in improvised coverings made of canvas or similar materials.

The hands and feet must be kept constantly warm and dry. For keeping the hands warm heavy woolen inner mitts with canvas or other windproof outer mitts are recommended.

Many a serious accident has occurred from touching cold metal with a bare hand. The metal will freeze to the skin. In the first reaction the tendency is to tear the hand away from the metal; this will destroy the skin. The metal should be thawed loose from the skin.

The Eskimo diet has been planned in relation to cold. Fat is the basis of this diet, for it is a heat-producing food. The Arctic soldier obtains his food from animals and fish. A government agency warns against the eating of polar-bear livers, which are said to be poisonous. Warning is also given against living exclusively on the meat of the rabbit, just because it happens to be plentiful. A continued diet of rabbit produces a condition called *rabbit starvation,* with diarrhea beginning about a week after the rabbit diet has been established. Practically all fish have enough fat to make them good Arctic food. The liver of the cod, which is the basis of cod-liver oil, is an especially good food and can be eaten boiled.

Among the most important of the recommendations are those having to do with the avoidance of *frostbite.* Frostbite often comes without the victim's knowledge. If the skin becomes stiff and grayish or whitish in color, frostbite is under way. Under such circumstances never apply snow or ice. This used to be the recommended treatment. Now we know that it is much better to warm the affected part gradually, avoiding even the gentlest of rubbing or massage, since this may destroy human tissue. Frozen feet are especially serious. If the feet are frostbitten, shoes and coverings should be removed immediately; when possible, a warmer type of footgear should be employed. The feet should be wrapped in cloth or fur until they thaw. Thawing is accompanied by a burning sensation and may be an extremely painful condition. After frostbite the skin blisters and peels exactly as it does in sunburn. *See also* CHILBAINS; FROSTBITE; GANGRENE; SKIN.

ARGYROSIS, a form of gray-blue discoloration of the skin and mucous membranes which results from deposits of silver particles. It is produced by the prolonged use of silver solutions, like *silver nitrate* or *Argyrol.*

ARM, in anatomy, the upper extremity of the body, from shoulder to elbow. Popularly, however, it indicates the arm and forearm.

ARTERIOSCLEROSIS, hardening of the arteries, a disease fairly common among older people. The walls of the blood vessels are clogged by depositions of minerals and fatty material and degenerate, losing their original resilience, and become thicker, tough, and more rigid. Arteriosclerosis represents from 25 to almost 50 per cent of all chronic circulatory disease, and is responsible for many deaths among persons living past middle age.

A healthy blood vessel can be compared to a hose made of elastic material. When the volume of liquid flowing through the hose is increased, the hose stretches to accommodate it, and when the volume of liquid decreases the hose shrinks. This is exactly what a healthy blood vessel does, stretching and shrinking to accommodate the increasing or decreasing volume of blood flowing through it. But when the walls of a blood vessel become rigid and inflexible, as in arteriosclerosis, this accommodation does not take place and when increased quantities of blood flow through a hardened or sclerotic artery, the pressure within the blood vessel rises temporarily, sometimes to the bursting point.

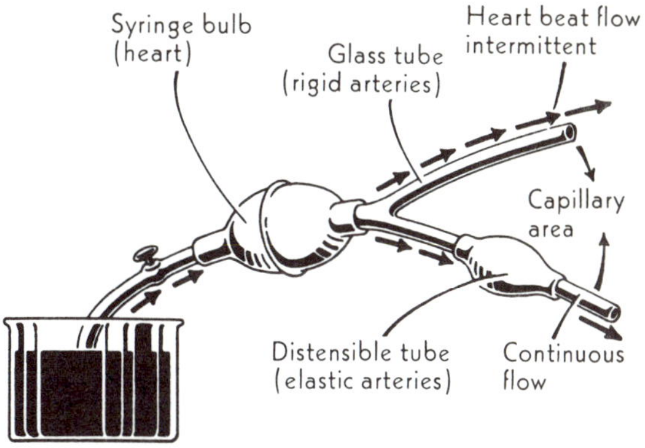

Arteriosclerosis — Mechanism showing how hardened blood vessels increase blood pressure. Normal blood pressure is dependent on many factors. Primarily, the energy of the heart action and the elasticity of the walls of the arteries influence pressure. Inelastic or rigid arteries interfere with the proper flow of the blood, build up pressure and force the heart to pump harder.

Actually the symptoms of hardened arteries develop largely from the effects of this condition on the blood pressure and the circulation of local areas of the body. Generalized high blood pressure throughout the body is not caused by hardening of the arteries, although the two conditions tend to be closely related.

The commonest symptoms of hardened arteries are drowsiness, periods of giddiness, headaches, and other manifestations of high blood pressure. Interference with circulation may cause cramps in the legs, which give them a bluish tinge. The most serious form of arteriosclerosis occurs when the blood vessels of the brain and heart are involved.

The specific causes of the hardening process within the arteries is not as yet fully understood and is the subject of much medical research.

the disease and its causes Arteriosclerosis is the name given to the loss of elasticity and the hardening of the arteries of the body. It occurs at all ages but is more truly a degenerative disease, affecting people in the older age group as their bodies begin to wear out.

Some men and women have an inherited tendency toward this illness, but it is more likely to be severe in patients with diabetes, sluggish thyroid, and those with high blood cholesterol. Most frequently it affects the arteries supplying blood to the brain, the extremities, and the heart. The aorta (the major artery supplying the body) is also frequently involved.

Cholesterol, saturated fats, and particularly excessive intake of refined carbohydrates such as sugar are believed to play an important role in the development of this disease. Certain diets raise blood cholesterol, cause fat to be deposited on the inner wall of the arteries, and hasten the clotting of blood. Thus, the formation of blood clots may be related to both the arteriosclerosis and the blood changes caused by diets rich in cholesterol. It would seem that diet is important both as a cause and a preventive in the most important form of arteriosclerosis–that involving the primary arteries.

symptoms When the disease is generalized there may be few or no symptoms. Symptoms of the extremities are illustrated in the Medi-Graph. When the brain is involved, there may be decrease in mental activity, loss of memory, dizziness, and confusion. Coronary arteriosclerosis, perhaps the most important form, results when the arteries feeding the heart become so narrowed that sufficient blood cannot get through.

complications Stroke, heart failure, gangrene of the legs, and the development of blood clots in the larger blood vessels of the body are possible complications.

prevention (or lessening of impact) Much can be done today to delay or control arteriosclerosis. Patients with a family history of high blood cholesterol or blood vessel disorders should be conscious of the importance of diet. They are urged to avoid the overuse of foods rich in refined carbohydrates, such as pies, cakes, and soft drinks, and concentrate on lean meat, fish, milk, and vegetable products. Smoking should be avoided. Exercise, as prescribed by the physician, should be a routine part of living. The doctor will also prescribe the proper thyroid extract for patients with hypothyroidism and high blood cholesterol. Any underlying disorder that might contribute to the development of arteriosclerosis should be treated promptly. In some cases, where the legs are involved, the diseased artery may be replaced surgically.

Vascular (blood vessel) diseases in diabetics are controlled where possible by treatment of the diabetes itself. For arteriosclerosis occurring without clear-cut contributing disorders, some drugs of limited effectiveness are available to moderate the disease.

Arteriosclerosis (Hardening of the Arteries)

Two Main Types of Arteriosclerosis

1. Hardening or Calcification

Unmarred Artery in Cross Section

A. Inner layer: smooth membrane to promote flow-through of blood

B. Middle layer: muscle that stretches to receive blood from heart, contracts to push blood along

C. Outer layer: fibrous coat that strengthens and protects inner layers

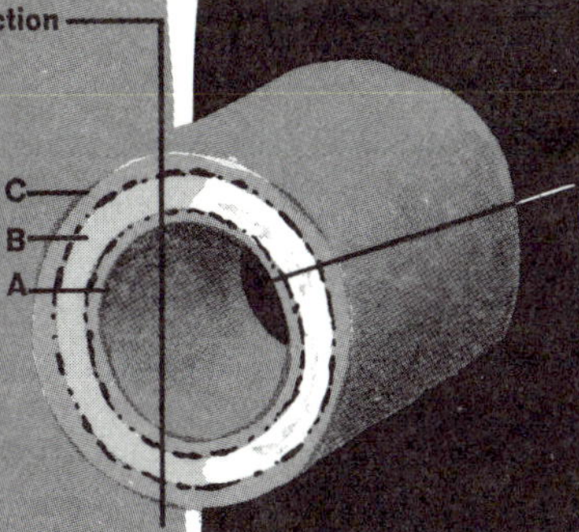

Middle layer fills with calcium—becomes hardened and brittle. But often does not narrow or obstruct blood flow. In these cases, not a dangerous condition

2. Arteriosclerosis

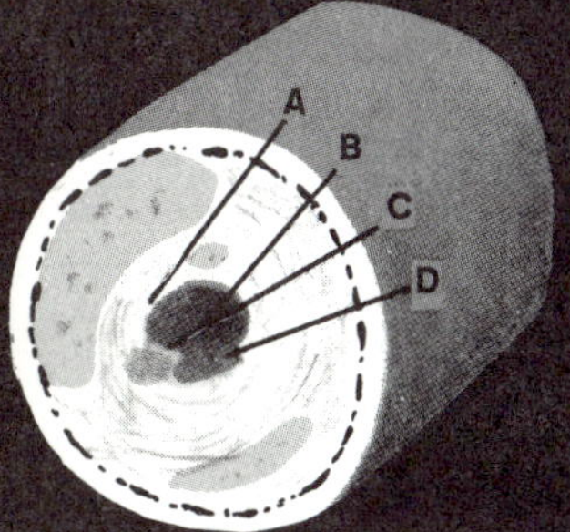

A. Deposits—mainly of cholesterol—build up on inner layer, thickening and roughening it
B. Thickening reduces the channel, cuts down easy flow of blood
C. Roughened surface promotes formation of blood clots—which further obstruct flow of blood
D. Thickening and roughening tend to go on progressively over the years

When arteriosclerosis attacks the body's major systems, other diseases may appear.

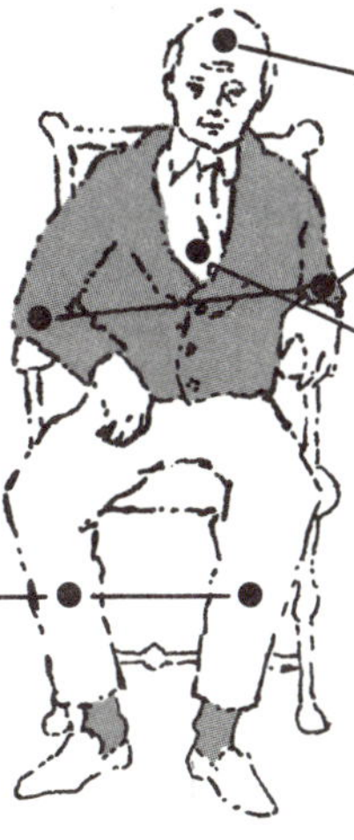

Central Nervous System: Stroke, paralysis of arms and legs

Central Heart-Blood Vessel System: High blood pressure, heart attack (coronary artery disease)

Outlying Blood Vessels: Gangrene of the legs (arteriosclerosis obliterans)

the disease and its causes In this illness the arteries to the legs become so narrowed that an insufficient blood supply passes through and the legs are deprived of essential nutrients. The causes are not completely understood, but the disease is considered a part of the aging process. Men are affected more often than women, and the disease occurs more frequently in patients who have diabetes.

symptoms The outstanding symptom is pain which occurs, as a rule, in the calves of the legs. When the patient exercises his legs, there is pain. When he rests, the pain disappears. This pattern of pain and rest is known as claudication. Usually the color of the leg involved is abnormal and it is cooler to the touch than the unaffected one. If the involved leg is elevated or exposed to cold, it turns pale. If it is warmed, it regains its color. If it is allowed to hang down after being elevated, it will first turn blue, and then red.

Often the patient complains of sharp shooting pains up and down the leg, particularly at night. The skin becomes very thin and shiny. A minor injury may cause it to ulcerate.

complications With the progression of the disease there are skin infections; brittle, slow-growing nails; and associated neuritic pain. In the final stages of a severe arteriosclerosis of the leg, gangrene may develop. Occasionally, osteomyelitis (an inflammation of the bone) results secondary to the infection. Amputation may be necessary.

prevention (or lessening of impact) There is no known preventive for peripheral arteriosclerosis. Patients should avoid smoking and take care not to become overweight. They should avoid injury and exposure to cold. An underlying disease such as diabetes should be adequately controlled. Foot care to avoid infection is most important. Athlete's foot and ingrown nails need particular attention. Once there is evidence of infection, energetic treatment should be employed. The physician will discuss with the patient who has peripheral arteriosclerosis various treatment techniques including nerve block, exercises, and surgery.

Peripheral Arteriosclerosis (Arteriosclerosis Obliterans)

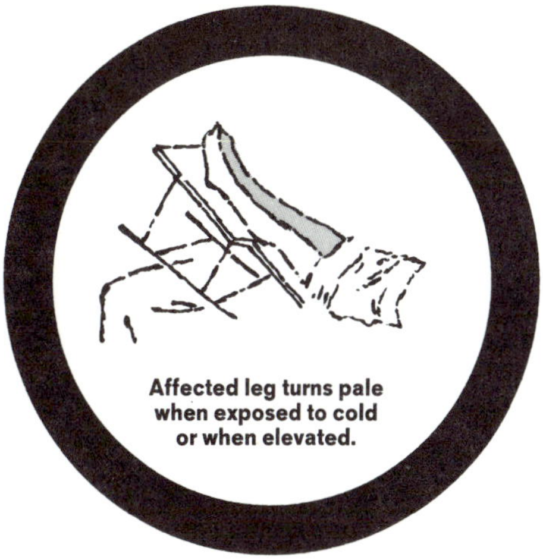

Affected leg turns pale
when exposed to cold
or when elevated.

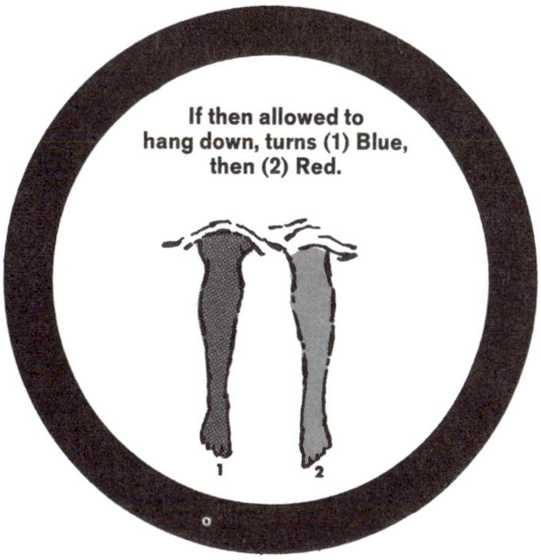

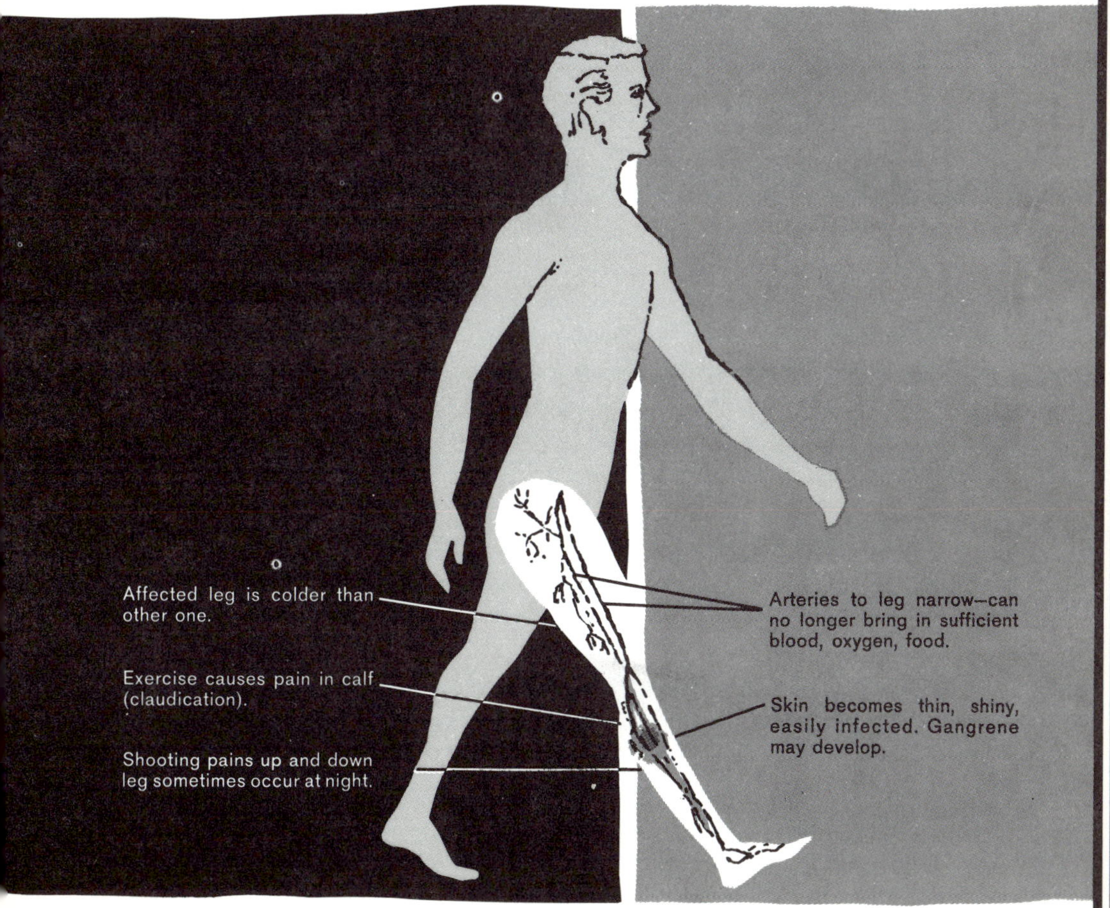

If then allowed to
hang down, turns (1) Blue,
then (2) Red.

Affected leg is colder than other one.
Exercise causes pain in calf (claudication).

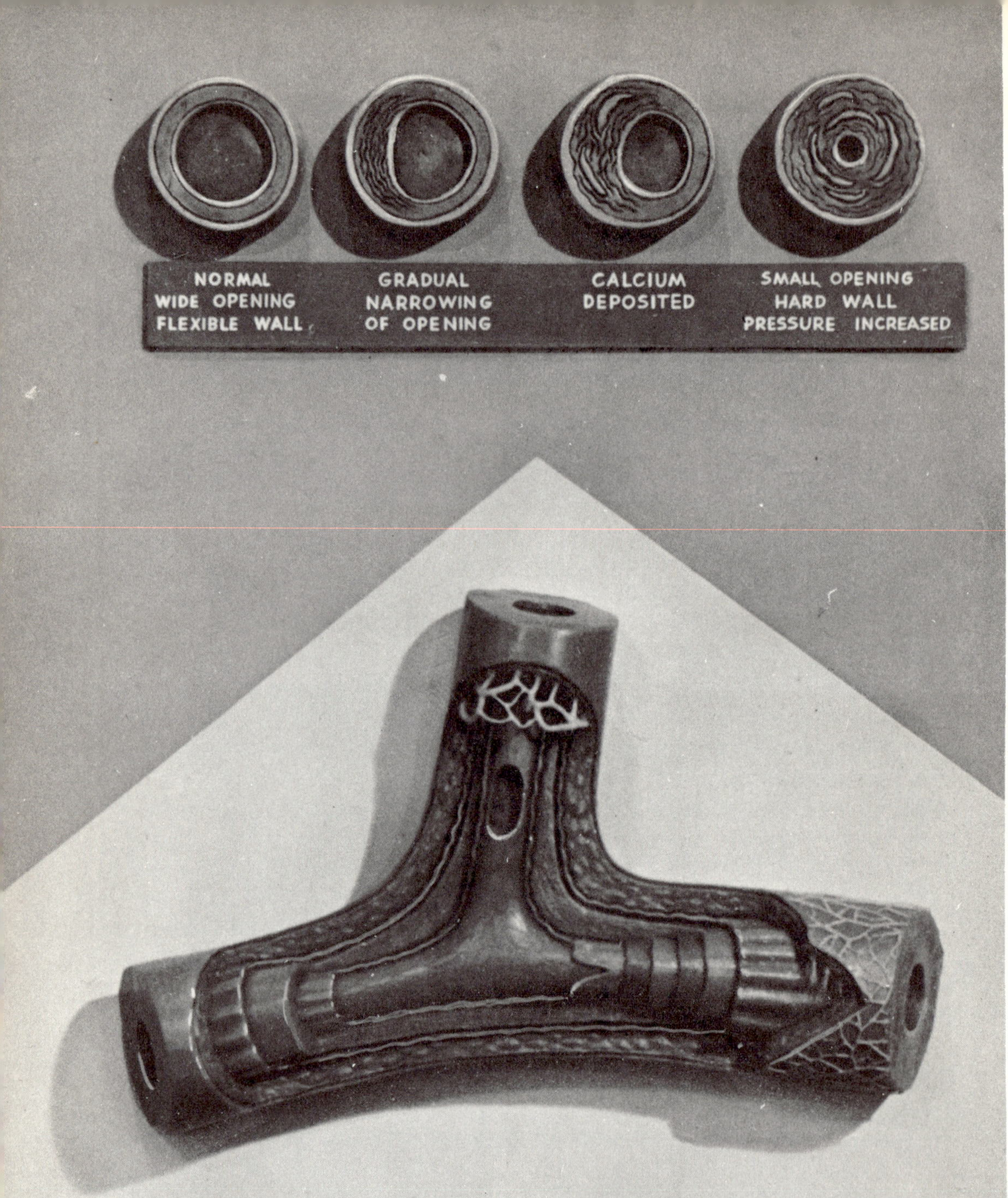

Arteriosclerosis—The large picture depicts the model of an artery, showing the various layers. In time, and as a result of certain diseases, minerals and fatty material are deposited in the wall making the artery narrow and stiff, thus causing high blood pressure. The small illustration at the top shows the gradual narrowing of an opening in the artery.

One theory, partly borne out by experimental work with animals, places responsibility on excessive consumption of fats. Another suggests that overindulgence of tobacco and alcohol somehow stimulate the condition, although this has never been proved scientifically. Still another attributes the onset of arteriosclerosis to excessive consumption of refined carbohydrates and sugars.

Treatment for arteriosclerosis is generally limited to establishing the patient's comfort and peace of mind as much as possible, and encouraging him to take good care of himself. The patient is urged to relax and eliminate as much as possible the stresses and strains of daily living, since excitement or intense emotion may stimulate a greater flow of blood than the hardened arteries can accommodate, with the possibility of severe consequences from rupture and bleeding. A low-fat diet is often recommended, and heat treatment, either baths or exposure to hot air, has been found useful. Several new drugs are available which often prove beneficial when prescribed. *See also* CIRCULATORY SYSTEM; APOPLEXY; CORONARY THROMBOSIS; FATS, UNSATURATED. *See* MEDIGRAPHS pages 229, 231, 371, 375, 697, 2233.

ARTERY. *See* CIRCULATORY SYSTEM.

ARTHRITIS, inflammation of the joints. Several million people in the United States are afflicted by various forms of arthritis, causing more days lost from work than any other disability except nervous and mental diseases.

Innumerable forms of inflamed joints affect people, and only a doctor can differentiate them. Arthritis may be caused by infection, by degeneration of joint tissues coincident with overweight or old age, or by deposits of uric acid crystals within the joint space, as in gout. Arthritis may follow injury or be associated with allergy to medicine or to food. Occasionally joint pain may indicate tumor growth or inflammation of the nerves surrounding a joint.

Arthritis due to infection of a joint resulting from tuberculosis, syphilis, typhoid fever, or gonorrhea is not as common now as in former years, because treatment of these diseases is now more effective. Joint pains due to allergy to penicillin or other drugs can be relieved by simple medications with antihistamines such as *Pyribenzamine, Benadryl,* or *Neohetramine.* Inflammation due to gout is treated by drugs such as *colchicine, Benemid, Butazolidin,* or *Anturan.* When the condition is caused by old injuries, surgery may occasionally be helpful in mollifying the scar tissue responsible for the pain. *Neuritis* and *neuralgia,* mimicking true arthritis, are sometimes relieved by large doses of the B vitamins.

Arthritis in women may be related to the function of the sex glands or ovaries. In postmenopausal arthritis, which occurs after

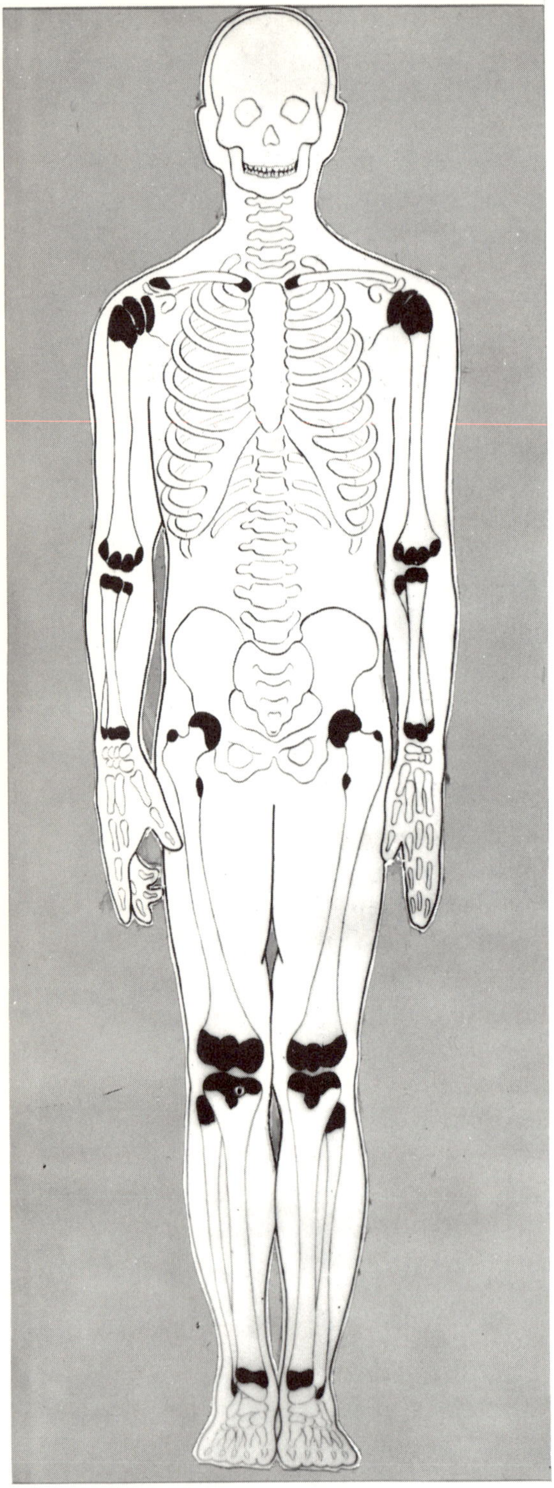

ovarian activity has ceased within the body, relief is often obtained with small doses of sex hormones.

Rheumatoid arthritis is somewhat more complex as well as more frequent than the types mentioned. While the exact cause is not known, certain factors have been established that definitely relate to the development of rheumatoid arthritis. Overfatigue, shock, injury, prolonged exposure to dampness or cold have all been thought to be associated with the development of this type of inflammation. Allergy has been postulated as a cause, as well as hormone defects. Rheumatoid arthritis often begins with a pain and stiffness in a single joint months before other joints become affected. It strikes the fingers, hands, wrists, and knees primarily, but may also affect the bones of the back and the hips. The fingers develop a typical "sausage-like" appearance in which the middle joint of the fingers becomes

Arthritis—The shaded areas on the ends of the bones show the linings of cartilage which reduce friction and are like bearings in the movable joints of the body. In some individuals, the joint cartilage does not sustain well under stress and strain and degenerative changes take place. Age, poor posture and joint injuries may also be contributing causes. The cartilage becomes thin and wears out. Bony growths develop from the surface of the bones, and the ends of the joint bones are in direct contact. Motion in the affected joint is limited and pain is present. The shoulders, end joints of fingers, spine, hips and knees are areas frequently involved in degenerative arthritis. Although cartilage cannot be replaced, relief of pain, heat, hydrotherapy, massage, rest, and a certain amount of exercise are valuable measures in treatment and in preventing further degeneration.

swollen and tender. The toes are seldom involved, as opposed to *gouty arthritis* in which the great toe is commonly affected. Nodules may occur under the skin in about 10 per cent of cases, usually located around the elbows, wrists, fingers, and occasionally the ankles. They vary in size from a small pea to a large walnut, appearing and disappearing without apparent cause.

Although true rheumatoid arthritis tends to be chronic, sudden complete relief of pain and stiffness may occur for months or years at a time. In mild cases the disability may be scarcely noticed, but in others the victim may become bedridden.

In older people, and in younger ones who are extremely overweight, *osteoarthritis* or *degenerative arthritis* may occur. The average age of onset of this type is between fifty and seventy, whereas rheumatoid arthritis usually strikes before forty and may affect children. In osteoarthritis the signs of inflammation are few. The symptoms of pain and disability are due to degeneration or wearing away of cartilage within the joint and, unlike rheumatoid arthritis which may affect almost any joint, the knees, back, and neck are most commonly involved. Swelling may occur in the last joint of each finger, but nodes are not found under the skin. Whereas rheumatoid inflammation tends to produce permanent deformity of the joints, osteoarthritis usually does not.

Many effective drugs and treatments are now available for persons afflicted with arthritis, depending on the particular type. For those suffering from rheumatoid arthritis, the discovery of *cortisone* has been most encouraging. With the help of this drug, former cripples are able to lead active lives. Use of this hormone, isolated from the *adrenal glands,* followed the observation that pregnant women often are completely relieved of arthritis during pregnancy. Dr. E. C. Kendall of the Mayo Clinic attempted to discover which element in the blood stream of pregnant women might be responsible for remission symptoms, and so cortisone was discovered. The results are often dramatic. Patients with severe rheumatoid arthritis may be relieved of pain and disability within a short time. Another and more potent form is *prednisone* (*Meticorten, Sertane* or *Del-*

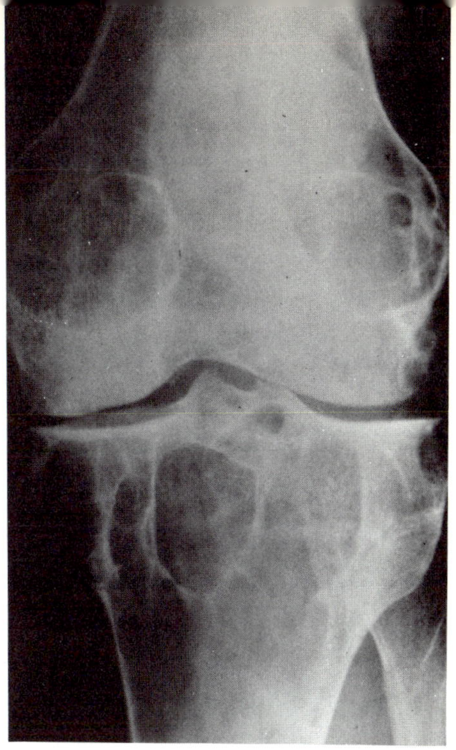

Arthritis—X-ray of bones in a joint of a rheumatoid arthritic patient, showing development of bone cysts.

Rheumatoid Arthritis

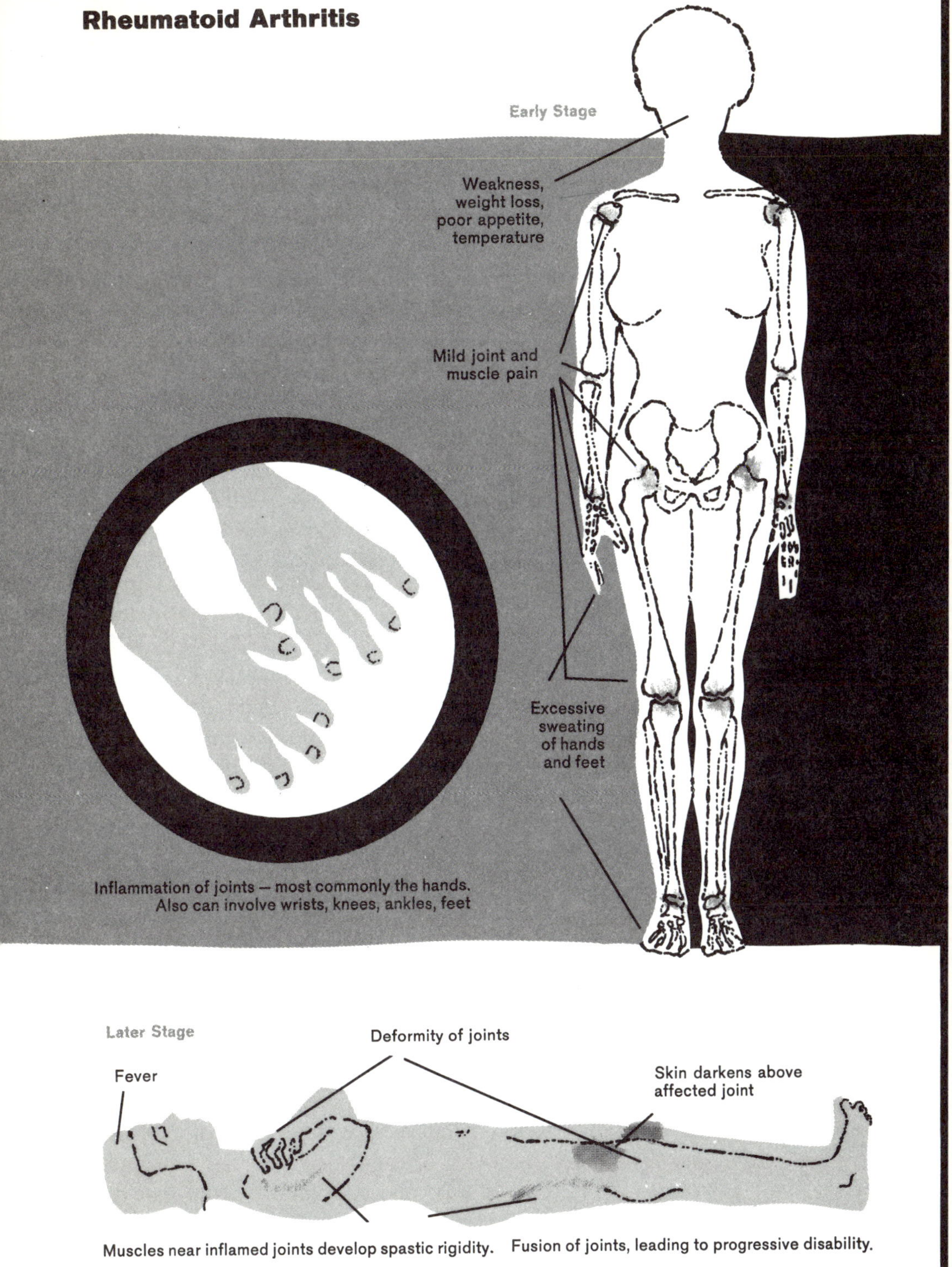

Early Stage
Weakness, weight loss, poor appetite, temperature
Mild joint and muscle pain
Excessive sweating of hands and feet
Inflammation of joints — most commonly the hands. Also can involve wrists, knees, ankles, feet
Later Stage
Deformity of joints
Fever
Skin darkens above affected joint
Muscles near inflamed joints develop spastic rigidity.
Fusion of joints, leading to progressive disability.

tra). *ACTH,* isolated from the *pituitary,* is another dramatically effective substance.

Unfortunately cortisone and ACTH do not *cure* arthritis. They do *relieve* disabling symptoms. These drugs must be taken indefinitely, always under the supervision of the attending physician. Although the drugs were originally quite expensive, newer techniques of producing cortisone may soon make arthritis treatment relatively inexpensive.

Rest is essential for the patient with arthritis. While he can continue to work, he should rest for an hour or two, preferably lying down after lunch. In severe cases, hospitalization may be necessary.

Diet may be significant. Patients are advised to eat a well-balanced, high-vitamin, high-protein diet, rich in vegetables and fruits.

Vaccines have been developed which are supposed to be useful. They are usually made out of bacteria that are isolated from the body of the person concerned, particularly from the nose, throat, and bowel. Their use seems to be still experimental. A number of patients are reported to have been benefited by such treatment. Many, however, feel that the effect of these vaccines is the same as comes from using a non-specific protein to stimulate the reaction of the body of the patient against any kind of infection. Occasionally, *blood transfusions* give relief.

The use of the *heat cabinet,* which produces artificial fever, has been reported to benefit some patients but there seems to be no evidence that it is routinely helpful. Such relief as occurs seems to be just temporary.

Frequently used remedies are *salts of gold.* There are several preparations of gold salts which are now tried and apparently anywhere from 20 to 40 per cent of patients report improvement when this treatment is given by a physician who has thorough knowledge of the technique of use of these preparations.

Reliance is especially placed on treating arthritis with *dry heat, diathermy, massage,* and *exercises,* in order to increase circulation to the joints, which may help retard the arthritic process and keep the surrounding muscles from becoming distorted or weakened. Many arthritis sufferers get considerable relief with *hot wet compresses. Aspirin, salicylic acid,* and *mild sedatives* are also beneficial in relieving arthritic pain, especially in milder cases that do not require cortisone. People with rheumatic ailments feel better in warm dry climates, such as those of Arizona and New Mexico. Wet damp environments may aggravate the condition.

Orthopedic surgeons can do much to improve the control of deformed bones and muscles in arthritis resulting from any cause. This, plus the amazing advances made in the medical care and treatment of arthritis, should brighten the hopes of everyone who suffers from this disease. *See also* GOUT. *See* MEDIGRAPHS pages 237, 1719.

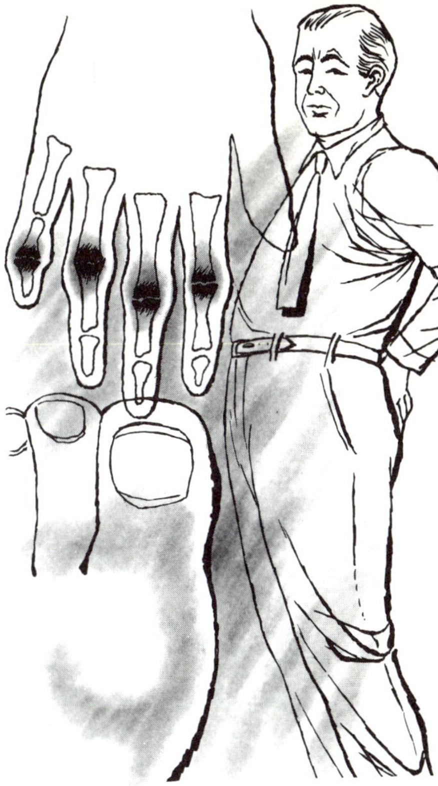

Arthritis, Rheumatism, and Gout

HOWARD F. POLLEY, M.D.

ARTHRITIS, RHEUMATISM, and gout are among the oldest diseases known to affect human beings. Hippocrates, a Greek physician called the "Father of Medicine," described these conditions graphically many centuries ago. Evidence of the occurrence of these diseases even before his time has been found in mummies and excavations from other ancient civilizations. The widespread occurrence of these diseases in the United States at present is indicated by the presence of some form of rheumatic disease in more than 16,500,000 people in this country.

The terms "arthritis" and "rheumatism" have been used synonymously at times, but as a result of advances in our medical knowledge, physicians have been able to recognize almost a hundred different kinds of arthritis and almost another hundred kinds of rheumatism. Arthritic diseases are those that affect singly or in various combinations the tissues of the joint: (1) the *cartilage,* (2) the adjacent *bone,* and (3) the *synovial* (*lining*) *membrane*. Rheumatism, by contrast, affects tissues *outside* the joint, sometimes spoken of as "the soft tissues." These tissues include the fibrous tissue which forms a capsule immediately surrounding the joint and also lines or envelops bundles of muscles and sheaths of nerves, ligaments, tendons, and bursae. Terms such as "fibrositis," "tendinitis," "bursitis," "myositis," or "myalgia," depending on which structure is affected, or the term "periarthritis," meaning around but not in the joint itself, may be used in describing the location of the rheumatism. Rheumatism may affect a person who also has arthritis, but rheumatism can and often does occur without arthritis.

There are both acute and chronic types of rheumatism and arthritis. Persons of any age and either sex may have practically any of the various types of arthritis and rheumatism. The most common type of arthritis is known as degenerative joint disease or *osteoarthritis,* which can be found to some extent in almost all persons past middle age. Hence this type of arthritis is often attributed to the results of "wear and tear" of use of joints of the body over a long time. Fortunately, though most persons may acquire some evidence of osteoarthritis, symptoms from the presence of the osteoarthritis occur only infrequently. Hence the presence of osteoarthritis is not necessarily evidence that a person's "rheumatic" or "arthritic" symptoms are the result of this type of arthritis.

Another type of arthritis of particular significance is *rheumatoid arthritis.* Physicians find that about one out of three patients who have symptoms of arthritis have this type of arthritis. It can affect persons of any age but tends to occur more commonly in the young adult years. Women are affected by rheumatoid arthritis two or three times as frequently as are men.

The most common types of rheumatism include *bursitis, fibrositis, tendinitis,* or *periarthritis* in the various parts of the body in which these tissues are particularly subject to rheumatic involvement. Another kind of rheumatism that is common is that which results from muscular and nervous tension and emotional fatigue. This is sometimes called *neuromuscular* or *psychosomatic rheumatism.*

Gout is a special type of metabolic disorder of the bodily functions which may be manifested by the occurrence at various times of either arthritis or rheumatism. Gouty arthritis (or bursitis or rheumatism) is related to the body's overproduction of or inability to dispose properly of chemicals, known as purines, eaten in certain foods or accumulating (as urates or uric acid) as a result of certain metabolic processes within the body itself. Gout usually affects men past middle age, although occasionally it occurs earlier than this. Gout affects women only infrequently (about one case in fifty), and then usually late in life. Gouty involvement occurs in the region of the "bunion joint" of the great toe, other joints of the feet, the ankles, and occasionally the knees, hands, wrists, or elbows. Usually only one joint or tendon or bursa is affected at a time. Attacks of gouty arthritis develop rapidly, and the affected area becomes red, warm, and extremely painful. The acute episode may last for a few days or perhaps weeks before it completely subsides. Even after the acute attack is gone, however, the basic derangement of bodily metabolism continues to exist and may require treatment. If the disease continues uncontrolled, multiple joints or articular areas may be affected and there may be gouty deposits in the bone and joints or bursae or ligaments which may be affected. This ultimately can result in a change from an acute to a chronic gouty arthritis. Similar gouty deposits are sometimes found on the ears, about the involved joints, and also in the kidneys. Patients with gout often have increased amounts of uric acid (as urates) in their blood, but such increases occur under a number of other circumstances. A test that shows an elevated concentration of uric acid in blood, of itself, therefore, does not necessarily indicate the presence of gout. Treatment for gout may include a special diet and drugs. This is discussed under the heading "Treatment of Arthritis, Rheumatism, and Gout."

CAUSES OF ARTHRITIS AND RHEUMATISM

Arthritis and rheumatism, like diseases of other organs of the body, can result from a number of causes, some known and others as yet unknown. These include (1) injury, (2) heredity, (3) infections, (4) allergies, (5) tumors, (6) metabolic disorders, and (7) fatigue, emotional upsets, or other factors.

INJURY

Injury to joints or related soft tissues may be either acute such as might be encountered in a fall, an automobile accident, or in the course of strenuous sports, or chronic injury such as that which might result from less severe but repeated daily injuries, such as those resulting from certain occupations or from other disadvantageous use over and over again of a certain joint or related musculoskeletal tissues.

HEREDITY

Arthritis and rheumatism can be produced by hereditary influences. The occurrence of a peculiar but common type of osteoarthritis in end joints of the fingers, called "Heberden's nodes," is an example of hereditary or familial development of osteoarthritis. The arthritis of the hemophiliac or "bleeder" is another example; this is more serious but fortunately is not common.

INFECTIONS

Arthritis and rheumatism can result from a number of different types of infections, including streptococcal and staphylococcal infections, pneumonia, meningitis, tuberculosis, venereal diseases, typhoid fever, undulant fever, and many others. Because of the infections which occur predominantly in children, certain types of infectious arthritis and rheumatism occur more frequently in younger than in older persons. Despite intensive investigations and long search, no germ or virus has been found to be the cause of osteoarthritis or rheumatoid arthritis.

ALLERGIES

Allergic reactions, or perhaps more properly reactions of hypersensitivity, may affect tissues involved by rheumatism or arthritis. Unusual sensitivity to drugs or proteins "foreign" to the human body, for example, may result in arthritis or rheumatism. When this type of arthritis or rheumatism occurs, it can be described as an inflammation without an infection.

TUMORS

Like other organs of the body, the joints may be affected by new growths or tumors, but fortunately these are rarely encountered in persons who have arthritic and rheumatic diseases.

METABOLIC DISORDERS

Changes in metabolism or the way in which the body performs its work may affect the joints and related skeletal tissues, thus resulting in arthritis or rheumatism. A severe deficiency of vitamin C, for example, may result in a disease called "scurvy" in which there may be rheumatic complications. A disorder in the body's ability to handle the purine (a type of protein) substances formed during certain metabolic processes or contained in certain foods results in the condition known as gout, which has been described. Ochronosis, a peculiar type of degenerative joint disease, occurs in some persons in whom pigmented chemical deposits develop in cartilage as a result of a particular abnormality of the body's enzymes. Similarly, a disturbance or upset of the balance between the various hormones of the body may affect the condition of joints or result in certain types of rheumatism or arthritis.

OTHER FACTORS CAUSING ARTHRITIS AND RHEUMATISM

Some physicians have suspected from time to time that arthritis and rheumatism may result from disturbances of circulation or disturbances of function of the nervous system. Lowered physical resistance, emotional upset, stress, shock, fatigue, and the like are other factors which might be of considerable importance to the development of certain types of arthritis and rheumatism.

In general, climate is neither a cause of nor a cure of arthritis or rheumatism. A few specific types of arthritis and rheumatism may be related to certain climates or geographical areas, but people in all parts of the world can and do have many of the common types of arthritis and rheumatism.

SYMPTOMS OF ARTHRITIS AND RHEUMATISM

Persons with arthritis and rheumatism often have a background of acute or chronic stress or strain. This may be of either a physical or mental nature or both and may be an important indication which will permit early recognition of the symptoms of articular or rheumatic diseases. Sometimes the first symptom is not directly related to the joints, but is more in the form of tiredness or exhaustion or generalized aching and stiffness. There may be loss of weight, appetite, and strength. The sensation of swelling of joints or muscles may be recognized by the person affected even though it may not be detected by careful examination of the affected areas. As would be readily recognized, these symptoms of a more or less general nature are not always indicative of arthritis or rheumatism. A person with such symptoms should rely on the advice and judgment of his physician in evaluation of these symptoms.

The main symptoms of arthritis or rheumatism are pain, stiffness, limitation of motion, and swelling of affected areas. Pain from arthritis and rheumatism varies from dull to sharp in severity, or may be described as "like a toothache" or "knifelike." In some types of rheumatism burning sensations and feelings of "pins and needles" and numbness may occur in affected areas. The pain may be fleeting or constant and may vary from one location to another or may occur only in an isolated area. The affected area may be warm or hot to touch, and there may or may not be some degree of redness or discoloration of the overlying skin. Pain of arthritis and rheumatism is often characterized by its "ups and downs," but may disappear without returning or may progress either slowly or fairly rapidly.

Patients with rheumatism and arthritis often complain of "stiffness." When rheumatic stiffness is aggravated by rest, it is often relieved by mild exercise and easy movements of the affected areas. When the stiffness is more directly related to fatigue, it may be relieved by rest and inactivity.

Limitation of motion of an affected area may result from pain on motion and consequent avoidance of that painful motion or may be related to muscular weakness or imbalance in muscular function. Sometimes limited motion also is attributed to fatigue. In other instances roughening of the smooth, shiny, cartilaginous surfaces of the joint may be the basis for limitation of motion. Creaking noises or crepitation on motion may also result from such changes in the joint surfaces, but the creaking sounds may be produced just as readily by friction in tissues outside the joint. Hence such sounds do not necessarily indicate that a joint is damaged or even diseased.

Swelling may occur either outside the joint or inside the joint. Swelling outside the joint often can be attributed to generalized fatigue or disturbances in the balance of function in small blood vessels which become "sluggish" in their capacity to remove or circulate the body fluids. Swelling of this type may produce the sensation of rings becoming temporarily tight on fingers or shoes tight on the feet. This type of swelling may occur either after periods of rest and inactivity or in parts of the body that are dependent or hang down during much of the time that a person is not resting.

Swelling that occurs inside the joint results from the collection of fluid in the joint in an amount in excess of that normally produced by the lining (synovial) membrane for lubrication of the joint. This may occur with certain types of inflammation, infection, injury, or other disorders. Local heat or warmth outside the joint often accompanies the collection of excess fluid, although when excess fluid has been present for some time there may not be apparent local heat, warmth, or redness of the covering tissues.

TREATMENT OF ARTHRITIS, RHEUMATISM, AND GOUT

As is to be expected, the treatment of arthritis or rheumatism depends on the type of involvement present. To determine this a careful medical examination is usually needed. When a cause of arthritis or rheumatism such as infection, allergy, tumors, or metabolic deficiencies is found and can be corrected, the arthritis or rheumatism subsides.

When a removable cause of the arthritis or rheumatism cannot be found, treatment is generally directed toward helping the patient (1) improve the ability of his natural bodily functions to cope with the arthritis or rheumatism, and (2) (when needed) maintain as nearly normal joint function as is possible. Thus in the treatment of arthritis and rheumatism both the daily activities and the periods of rest need to be considered carefully; neither should the former be excessive nor the latter be minimized or slighted. Adequate rest and sound sleep, a mind free of worry and daily activities free of anxiety and tension go a long way toward improving the body's ability to cope with the presence of extra inflammation, infection, or other factors requiring special effort by the bodily functions. *How* well this is accomplished is generally more important than *where* it is done. The position of joints during resting hours should be favorable to use of the joints when rest is not needed. This is discussed in the following section on "Physical Therapy." An occupation that protects affected joints and muscles, minimizes fatigue and loss of bodily energy and resistance may be another means of improving the natural bodily resistance against arthritis or rheumatism.

It is sometimes advisable for persons who have arthritis or rheumatism to sleep in a warm room, wear warm socks, mittens, or a head covering, in addition to the bedclothes, or use an electric blanket. Whether any exposure to the sun is desirable is determined by the type of arthritis or rheumatism present. Such persons must rely on the advice of their physician regarding this matter as well as for advice concerning the amount of exposure to sun that is desired.

Extra care to protect against exposure to infections is usually desirable, especially when resistance is low or when fatigue is present. Attention to dental and other bodily hygiene also constitutes an important aspect of the general bodily care of the arthritic or rheumatic patient.

A well-balanced diet, including meat, vegetables, fruit, and dairy products, is usually advisable. The details of a normal diet have been presented in another chapter in this book. The physician can decide when dietary supplements (such as vitamins and iron) are indicated. Many dietary fads have appeared from time to time, but, in general, the arthritic or rheumatic person does best to eat the type of food which would be best for him if he were not troubled by arthritis or rheumatism. It is generally advisable for rheumatic and arthritic patients to avoid being overweight in order to provide additional protection to weight-bearing joints.

The diet for patients with gout and gouty arthritis may require restricted use of foods containing significant amounts of purine substances. Wild game and fowl, and meats derived from animal organs, such as liver, kidneys, sweetbreads, brains, and so on, contain large amounts of purine and are especially to be avoided. Certain other meats and meat extracts used in soups and gravies may be allowed in the diet, but amounts are generally restricted. Alcoholic beverages may be excluded from the diet, but coffee, tea, cocoa, milk, and fruit juices can be permitted. A person with gout can best determine his particular dietary requirements by detailed consideration of his individual needs with his physician or a dietitian instructed by the physician.

PHYSICAL THERAPY

Since efforts to improve a person's general physical condition may involve spending extra time in bed each day, special attention may need to be given to the maintenance of joint function that will be as useful as possible when the patient does not require rest. Pillows under knees or hands, and arms folded over the chest, for example, are positions usually to be avoided during resting hours. Judicious use of splints, sandbags, lightweight plaster or plastic casts, a board under the mattress of the bed, and other supportive measures, however, can be helpful in maintaining a desirable position. During the waking hours and when a person is up and about, strains or pressure on affected joints and soft tissues should be avoided. The additional support of various types of corsets, braces, properly supporting shoes, and other similar devices also can give some assistance. Even when joints have already been affected and *normal* function is not to be anticipated, it still may be possible to obtain some degree of *useful* function. This can be the difference between the person's being self-dependent, that is, in his being able to earn a living or care for a family, and not being able to do these things. Various types of physical therapy are available and can be used to help an arthritic or rheumatic person improve his condition as much as possible.

Heat and Massage

Heat in almost all forms is one of the helpful measures of physical therapy which most arthritic and rheumatic patients can use to good ad-

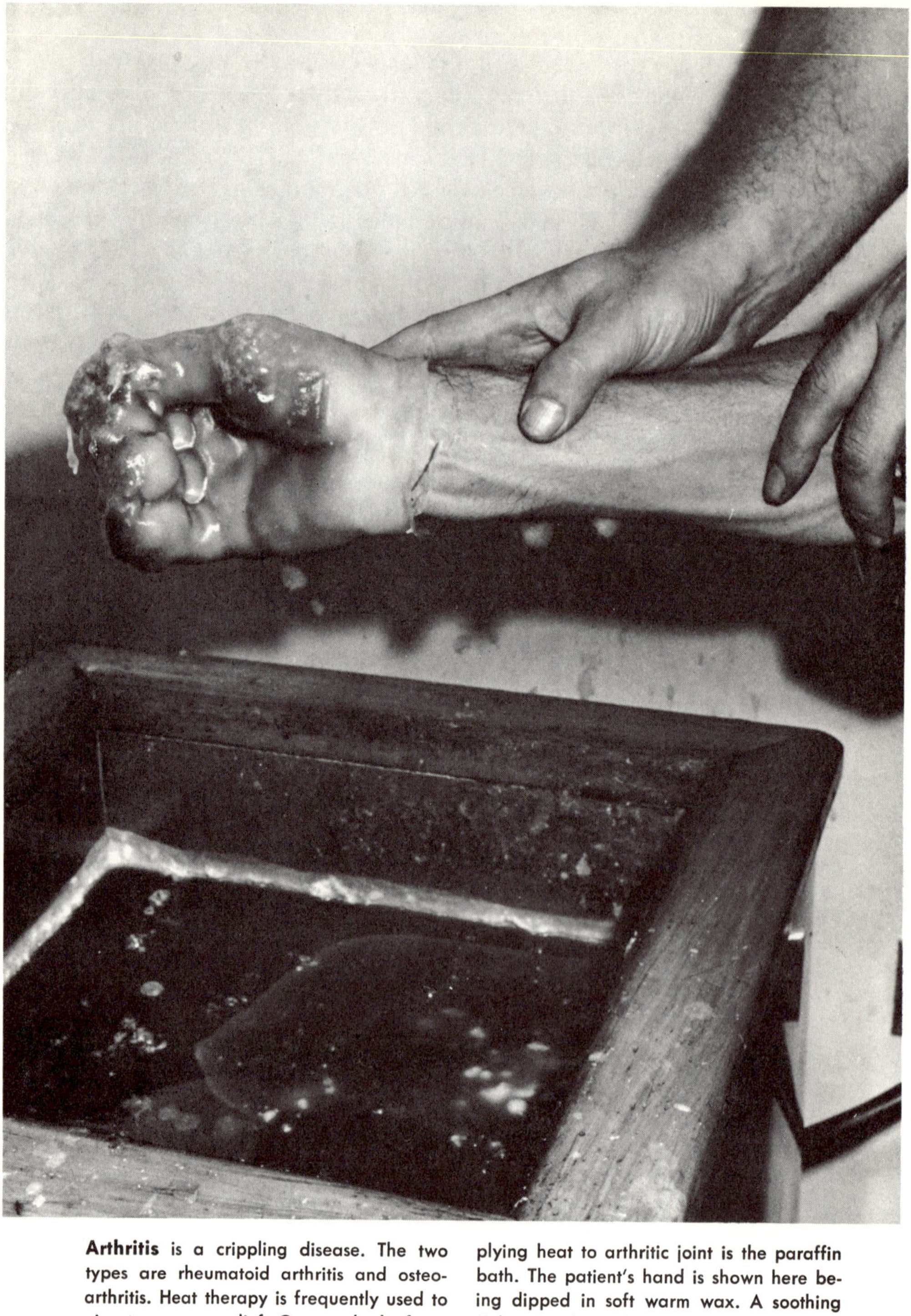

Arthritis is a crippling disease. The two types are rheumatoid arthritis and osteoarthritis. Heat therapy is frequently used to give temporary relief. One method of applying heat to arthritic joint is the paraffin bath. The patient's hand is shown here being dipped in soft warm wax. A soothing "glove" is formed.

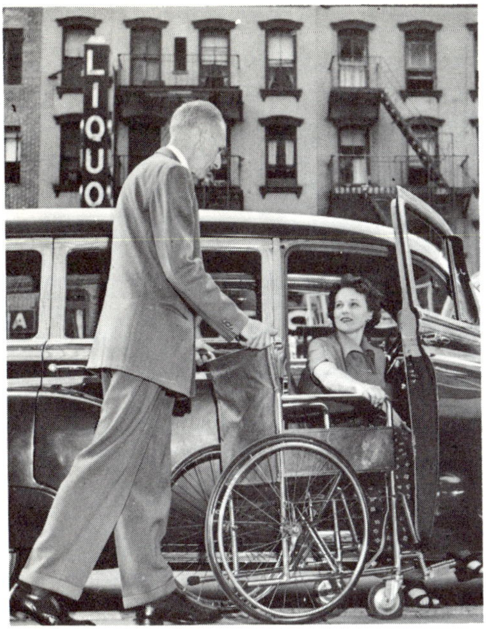

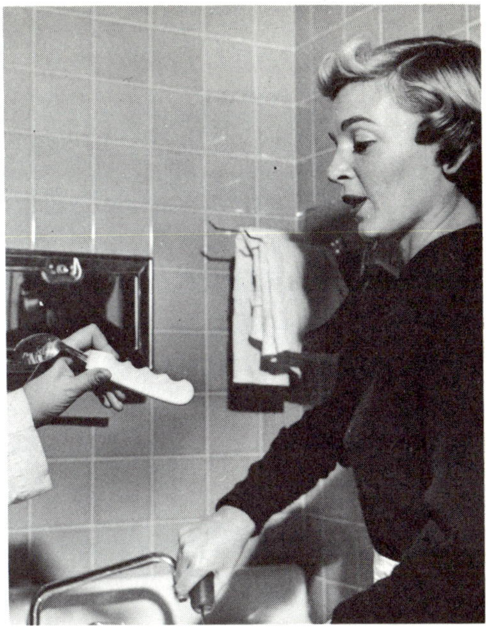

Special provision for transportation of the arthritic to place of treatment is often necessary. Specially designed equipment is of great assistance in manual tasks. An example is the spoon handle shown here. For patients with many arthritic joints, overall heat is administered in a large whirlpool unit, as shown below.

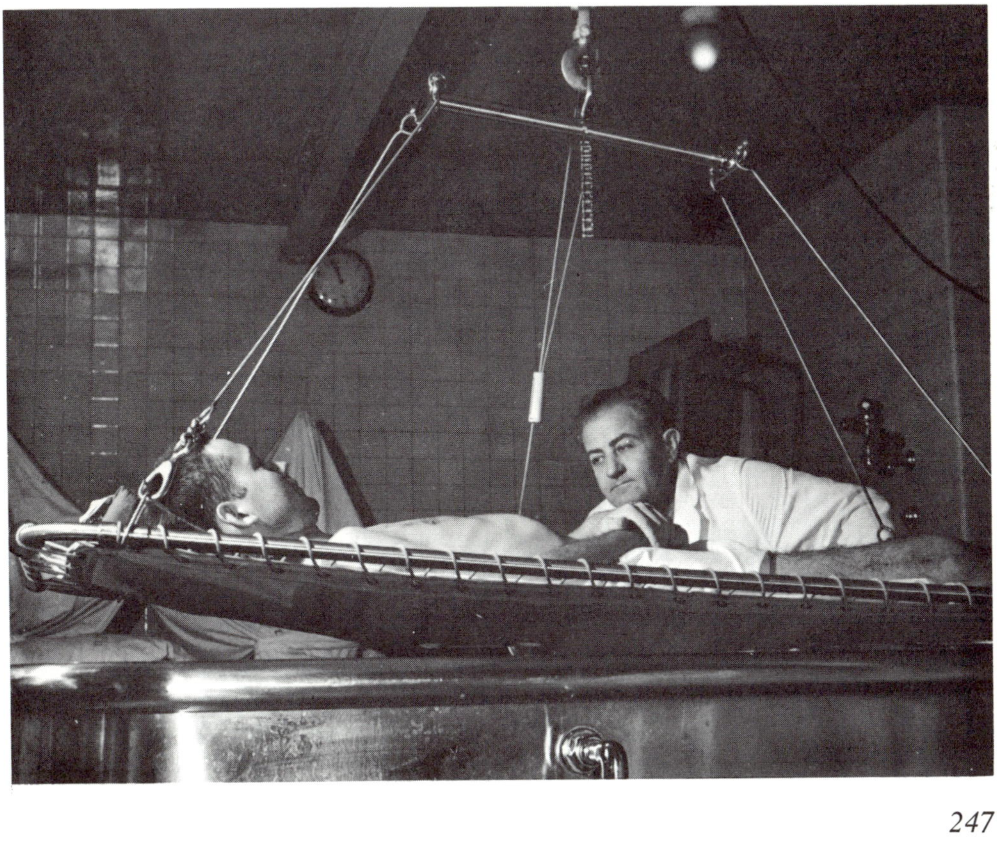

vantage. Occasionally, however, heat will not be indicated or will need to be used limitedly. Applications of heat increase the circulation and induce rest and relaxation in a painful muscle, joint, or other skeletal tissues. Many devices are available for the application of heat in the patient's home, including ordinary electric light bulbs, heat lamps and pads, warm tub baths, applications of warm or hot towels, woolen or flannel materials. Applications of paraffin and use of hot and cold contrast baths, when properly carried out, are other effective methods of utilizing heat. Care must be taken to avoid burns and overheating. It is advisable to consult a physician regarding the details of such treatment.

The application of heat is sometimes followed by massage performed under the direction of a physician or by either a trained physical therapist or a member of the patient's family who has been properly instructed in such treatment. The use of mechanical devices for massage may be hazardous and hence is not advised. The duration and type of massage vary with the type of rheumatism or arthritis, and specific instructions are also required for proper use.

Heat and massage, besides being of value in relieving symptoms of arthritis or rheumatism, also serve as a good preliminary to therapeutic exercise.

Therapeutic Exercise

The use of exercise as well as the type of such treatment which may be advisable is determined by the type of arthritis or rheumatism which may be present. "Therapeutic exercise" is designed to maintain or obtain as nearly normal strength, endurance, and range of motion in affected joints and muscles as it is possible to obtain. A person's ordinary daily activities rarely serve as a suitable substitute for therapeutic exercise, but when properly undertaken, therapeutic exercise, including postural and deep-breathing exercises, can be especially beneficial and should be performed daily. The conscientious application of the appropriate therapeutic exercises for whatever period of time they are needed constitutes one of the best approaches to the problem of how useful articular function may be regained or maintained in many types of arthritis and rheumatism. Therapeutic exercise should be undertaken only on the advice of a physician and when specific instructions regarding such treatment are made available. A physician may instruct a patient to use a pamphlet such as that prepared by The Arthritis Foundation, 1212 Avenue of the Americas, New York, New York 10036, or other supplements to supply additional information for effectively carrying out a program of home physical therapy.

TREATMENT WITH DRUGS AND OTHER MEASURES

Simple analgesics such as aspirin (acetylsalicylic acid) or closely related chemicals of the salicylate family are often of aid in giving relief from the pain of arthritis, rheumatism, or gout. Many highly advertised and ofttimes expensive patent remedies have utilized this beneficial effect by having the inexpensive salicylates as their principal effective ingredient. When a physician advises the use of aspirin or other salicylates, there should be no hesitancy on the part of the patient to use such treatment to best advantage. Of course, these drugs like many others are not to be used indiscriminately, but a popular opinion that such drugs are "bad for the heart," stomach, kidneys, or other organs is exaggerated, if not erroneous. Aspirin and other salicylate drugs can relieve painful spasm as well as counteract inflammation and are not "dope" or habit-forming drugs. However, for nearly all types of arthritis and rheumatism, narcotic drugs which can be habit-forming should be avoided. This is especially true when treatment for arthritis or rheumatism is likely to be prolonged.

For some severe inflammatory reactions other anti-inflammatory and immunosuppressive drugs which need to be used with appropriate medical supervision have become available.

For the special type of arthritis which patients with gout have periodically, a drug known as colchicine is of particular value. This time-tested remedy has been used successfully for more than a hundred years for acute gouty arthritis, but it usually is not of benefit to other types of arthritis or rheumatism. Drugs which either accelerate the elimination of excess uric acid from the body or interrupt internally its formation also often are needed to control gout.

Although it is not yet known just how the benefit is mediated, gold salts given by injection are sometimes helpful for persons with rheumatoid arthritis. Use of X rays, exposure to various radioactive materials, specially prepared or processed foods, blood transfusions, vaccines, or tonics has now been largely replaced by other types of treatment which are more likely to be of benefit. Operations to repair or reconstruct affected joints may reduce disability from certain types of arthritis. With new or better techniques, the results of such operations are continually being improved. The limitations of such treatment, however, add a further impetus to efforts to prevent whenever possible the development of disability which might require such operative treatment.

TREATMENT WITH HORMONES

Nearly all the hormones of the body which have been isolated have been tested for their value in the treatment of various types of arthritis and rheumatism. The most effective to date have been certain of the hormones of the adrenal gland, known as cortisone and hydrocortisone, and the hormone of the pituitary gland, corticotropin or ACTH, which stimulates the cortex or outer layer of the adrenal gland to produce these adrenal steroid hormones. Prednisone, prednisolone and a number of other synthetic "chemical relatives" of cortisone and hydrocortisone have been produced in recent years. The various chemical modifications which are available and the improvements in techniques of administration of all adrenal hormonal preparations have permitted more patients to tolerate and benefit from such treatment than was the case in the early years of this relatively new type of treatment. However, adrenal hormone therapy generally is restricted to those persons with rheumatoid arthritis, or certain closely related types of arthritis, which are not adequately controlled by other indicated treatments. Thus, treatment with an adrenal steroid hormonal preparation usually will *supplement* rather than be a substitute for other treatments which already have been discussed. To obtain the optimal and sustained advantages of hormonal treatment of rheumatoid arthritis, dosage needs to be highly individualized. This requires careful medical supervision of such treatment. However, when use of these hormones is advised by a physician familiar with them, a person may proceed with the same confidence and consideration he would have in accepting other types of treatment.

Treatment with adrenal steroid hormones may be carried out by using certain preparations that can be injected into the affected joint or joints or inflamed extra-articular tissues, but treatment with adrenal hormones is not advised for many types of arthritis and rheumatism, including the rheumatism from fatigue or nervous and emotional upsets, the arthritis of injuries, or the arthritis and rheumatism resulting from specific types of infections by germs. Injections of suitable steroid preparations may be made into the joints or extra-articular tissues of certain patients with degenerative joint disease or osteoarthritis, but adrenal steroids usually are not given systemically for this condition. Arthritic and rheumatic persons may reasonably anticipate that the further efforts of medical and chemical scientists will improve the physician's ability to affect the course of the various types of arthritis and rheumatism and gout.

RESULTS OF TREATMENT

Use of currently available methods of determining the type of arthritis or rheumatism and adequate application of currently available treatment will provide most patients with considerable comfort and useful joints. Success in treatment is a co-operative venture on the part of the patient and physician. Rarely can the physician facilitate the accomplishment of the objectives of treatment without the expenditure of much time and effort by the person affected.

ARTIFICIAL LIMBS, known also as *prostheses,* which means artificial substitution for missing parts such as legs, arms, and dentures. Improved prosthetic techniques have always followed wars. Today the stumps of limbs are being effectively used by salvaging the functions of the remaining muscles in the stump to manipulate the artificial replacements.

Many materials are suitable for the manufacture of artificial limbs. Wood, especially willow, has excellent qualities and is generally used. Aluminum, or duralumin has the advantage of lightness and is therefore preferable for weak and elderly people. Much work is being done with plastics but as yet is still largely in the experimental stage. The U.S. Army uses fiber in artificial limbs. The straps, belts, and foot coverings are made of leather, although it has certain disadvantages.

In artificially replacing a lower limb, the ankle and knee, and particularly their sockets, are especially important. The socket determines the gait. The amputee must learn to use the artificial limb effectively, which involves control of his thigh and hip muscles.

Because of its intricacy, the artificial arm is used less than the artificial leg. The type of replacement depends to a large degree upon the occupation of the amputee. Some find the peg arm, a stable jointless short arm, best since it can be fitted with a hook which gives great lifting power. The voluntary-control hand can hold a pencil and other small objects, and many utility appliances can be worn for special occupations, depending on the needs. A recent development is a hook operated by a chest or arm muscle. Through an operation known as *cineplasty* the control muscle is brought outside the body and covered by skin, and the device is then managed by contracting the muscle. Artificial hands that are purely cosmetic and without any functional purpose are also available.

ARTIFICIAL RESPIRATION. One of the basic first-aid measures is knowing how to restore natural breathing when drowning, suffocation, or some other accident has caused it to stop. The revised standard technique for artificial respiration, as approved by the American National Red Cross, is known as the mouth-to-mouth method of resuscitation. This is considered the best way of reviving infants and children whose breathing has stopped. It consists of the following steps:

1. Clear the mouth of foreign matter with the middle finger of one hand, and with the same finger hold the tongue forward.

2. Place the child in a face-down, head-down position, and pat him firmly on the back with the free hand. This should help dislodge any foreign object in the air passages.

3. Place the child on his back and use the middle fingers of both hands to lift the lower jaw from beneath and behind so that it "juts out."

4. Hold the jaw in this position, using one hand only.

5. Place your mouth over the child's mouth and nose, making a relatively leakproof seal, and breathe into the child with a smooth steady action until you observe the chest rise. As you start this action, move the free hand to the child's abdomen, between the navel and the ribs, and apply continuous moderate pressure to prevent the stomach from becoming filled with air.

6. When the lungs have been inflated, remove your lips from the childs' mouth and nose and allow the lungs to empty. Repeat this cycle, keeping one hand beneath the jaw and the other hand pressing on the stomach at all times. Continue at a rate of about twenty cycles a minute. If at any time resistance to breathing into the child is felt and the chest is felt and the chest does not rise, repeat second step, then quickly resume mouth-to-mouth breathing.

See also ASPHYXIA; DROWNING; RESUSCITATION.

ASBESTOSIS, a lung disease which occurs among workers who inhale dust and other materials from asbestos, a complex calcium magnesium silicate. Inhalation of asbestos fibers produces fibrous changes in the lungs which represent an attempt of the tissue of the lung to wall off the foreign substance.

Asbestos contains about 41 per cent iron oxide. The lungs react particularly to silica and develop *silicosis.* Workers with asbestos also develop warty growths, called *asbestos corns,* on the skin. *See also* INDUSTRIAL HEALTH; INHALING OF DANGEROUS SUBSTANCES; OCCUPATIONAL HAZARDS IN INDUSTRY.

ASCARID, a type of long cylindrical parasite worm which sometimes infests the intestines.

ASCHHEIM-ZONDEK TEST, a test for pregnancy in which the urine of the woman being tested is injected subcutaneously into immature female mice. A positive reaction is indicated by swelling, congestion and hemorrhages of the murine ovaries and premature maturation of the ovarian follicles. Named for Selmar Aschheim and Bernhardt Zondek, German gynecologists. *See also* TESTS.

ASCORBIC ACID, or vitamin C, a white or slightly yellowish crystalline powder, soluble in water, is an organic compound found in citrus fruits and juices, fresh green leafy vegetables like kale and broccoli, potatoes, cantaloupe, tomatoes, and strawberries. Ascorbic acid is essential to the proper development of teeth and bones and the walls of capillary blood vessels. It is an aid in resisting infection and its absence leads to the once dreaded *scurvy.* Vitamin C is significant in infant diet, and is usually added two weeks after birth. Children may need a supplementary form of this vitamin, but only on recommendation of a doctor. An adult requires 75 mg. daily. *See also* VITAMINS.

ASEPSIS, the absence of disease-producing bacteria. A wound is aseptic if it is cleansed and in germ-free condition. *See also* ANTISEPTICS.

ASPHYXIA, suffocation, coma or unconsciousness caused by deprivation of oxygen which results in accumulation of carbon dioxide and fixed acids. When breathing stops, no matter what the cause, oxygen must be supplied artificially or unconsciousness will take place, followed shortly by death.

The causes of asphyxia or suffocation are many, the most frequent being electric shock, gas poisoning, heart attacks, brain injuries, smoke, and drowning. Babies occasionally suffocate in their cribs.

Many industries and nearly all cities and towns have first-aid teams which can handle cases that require artificial respiration. Many different machines have been developed to aid resuscitation, and they are available at most fire departments, police emergency services, and hospitals. Ambulances are equipped with emergency apparatus to give aid to the victim of asphyxia at the earliest moment as well as during the ride to the hospital for further treatment. However, time must not be lost waiting for equipment to be brought to an asphyxiated person. Artificial respiration should be started immediately. Few people survive after their lungs have gone without a change of air for more than twelve minutes. In drowning, this time is reduced to four minutes.

A person who has drowned should be placed immediately in a horizontal position, back up, abdomen down, head turned to one side and resting on one hand to keep sand or water out of the mouth and eyes. If the body can lie slightly inclined downward on a slope of twenty to thirty degrees, elimination of fluid from the throat and the breathing tubes will be facilitated. Then alternate pressure and release on the chest is applied, forcing air in and out of the chest. Artificial respiration must be kept up, regardless of time, until medical help arrives.

A form of artificial respiration known as the back pressure-arm lift was formerly recommended by the American National Red Cross and was adopted in the armed services and other organizations. Here the victim is placed face down in a prone position, with arms overhead and bent at the elbows, one hand upon the other, and the head turned to one side so that the cheek rests on the hands. The rescuer, on one or both knees at the victim's head places his hands on the victim's back, with thumbs just touching, and the heels of the hands just below a line running between the victim's armpits. The rescuer rocks forward slowly, elbows straight, until his arms are almost vertical, exerting steady pressure upon the back. Next the rescuer rocks backward slowly and slides his hands to the victim's arms, just above the elbows, which are raised until resistance is felt at the victim's shoulders. Then the arms are dropped. This completes a full cycle, which is repeated twelve times a minute.

Most recently recommended is mouth-to-mouth artificial respiration, and when available use of a tube through which air is blown and exhaled. This tube also keeps the tongue out of the way.

Everything possible must be done to keep the asphyxiated person warm, because failure to do so may result in shock, which in turn may be responsible for death.

Linesmen working on electric wires are shocked and asphyxiated frequently and a special technique has been developed to meet such an emergency. As the shocked linesman is probably hanging by his safety belt, the rescuer pushes the victim's head forward and circles the waistline with his arms, placing one open hand on the abdomen and then grasping the first hand with the fingers of the other to insure a firm grip. Pressure is applied on the abdomen inward and upward, then completely released. The cycle is repeated, making about eighteen to twenty pressures a minute.

Rescucitation should be attempted for long periods of time, with the hope that the period during which the person has been without air is less than has been originally estimated. *See also* RESUSCITATION; DROWNING.

ASPIRATION, the act of breathing; may also indicate the removal of fluids or gases from a cavity by suction.

ASPIRIN. *See* ACETYLSALICYLIC ACID; MEDICINE CHEST, *Pain Relievers.*

ASTASIA, inability to stand in a normal manner because of lack of coordination. *Astasia-abasia* is a symptom of neurosis in which the affected person is apparently unable to walk or stand normally and seems to collapse when he tries to walk or stand.

ASTHENIA, lack of vitality and loss of strength which creates a general weakness. *See also* EXHAUSTION; FATIGUE; UNDERWEIGHT, HAZARDS OF.

ASTHENOPIA, weakness of the eye muscle and of visual power due to overuse or to errors of refraction. *See also* EYE.

ASTHMA, a disorder of the upper respiratory tract involving the lungs and the bronchi, characterized by wheezing, coughing, choking and shortness of breath. Asthma is a symptom and not a disease; therefore remedial measures involve locating, isolating and eliminating the cause rather than treatment of the condition itself.

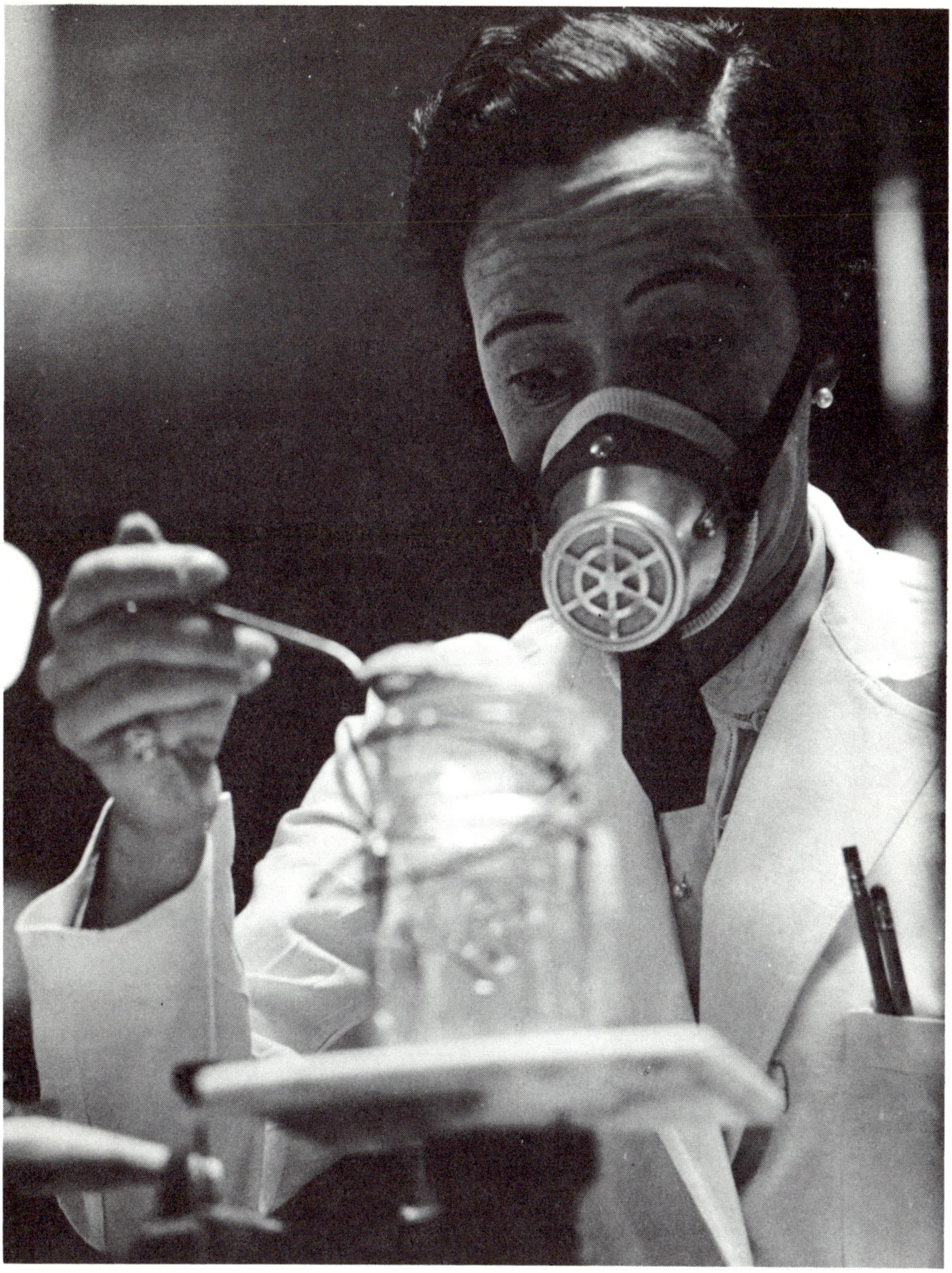

Asthma may result from an irritation to the respiratory system caused by a substance to which the victim is allergic. This may be dust, pollen, animal dander, certain foods, or even heat or cold. The cause can also be emotional. Above, a respirator enables the subject to handle pollen without any asthmatic reaction.

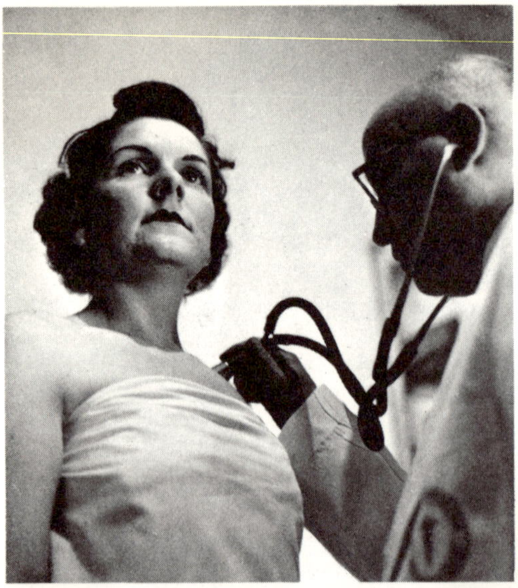

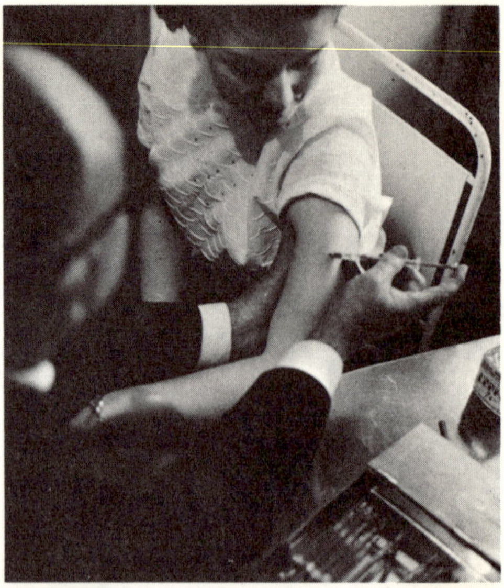

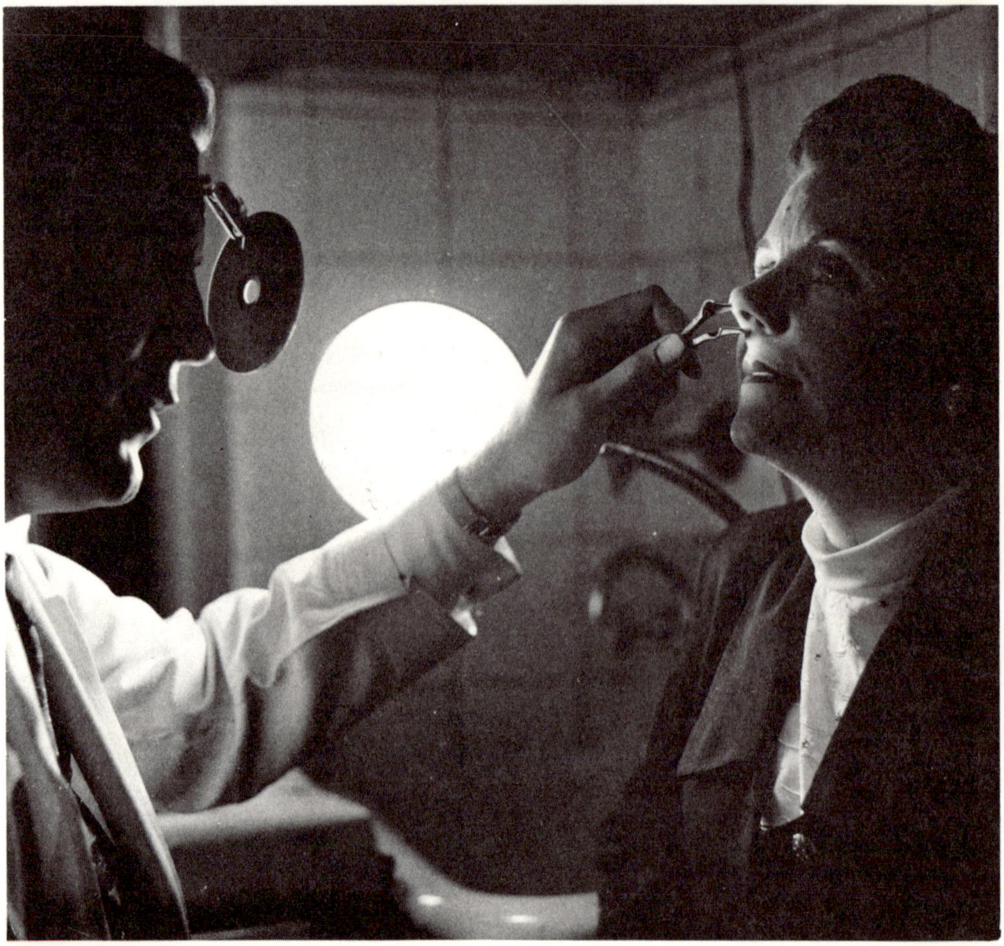

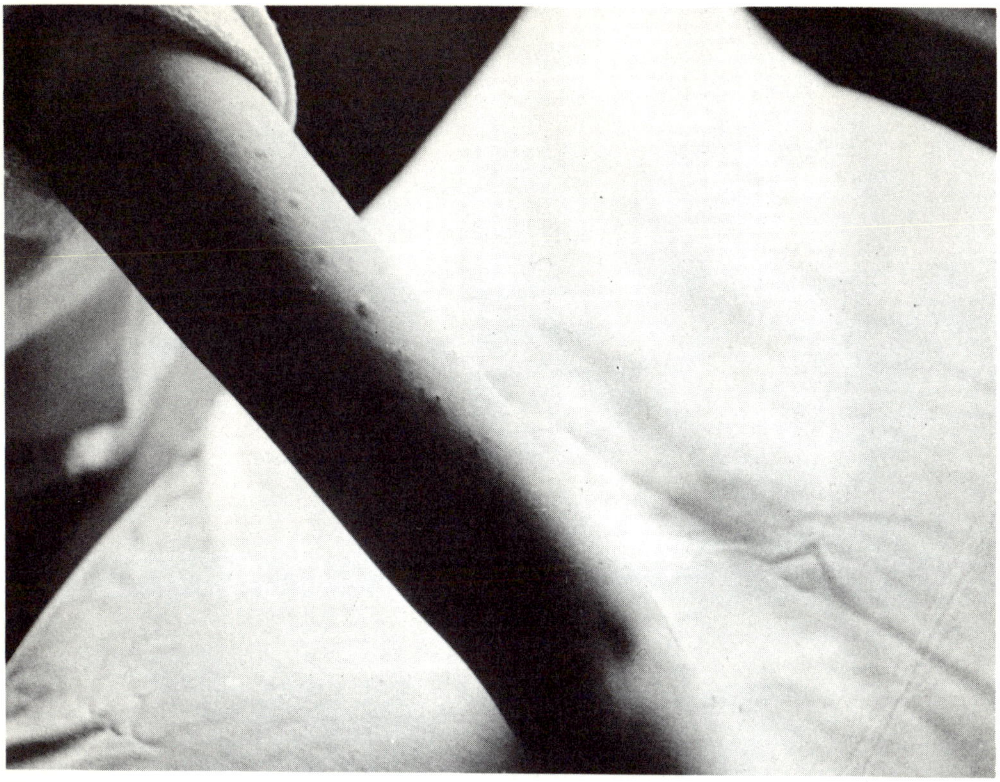

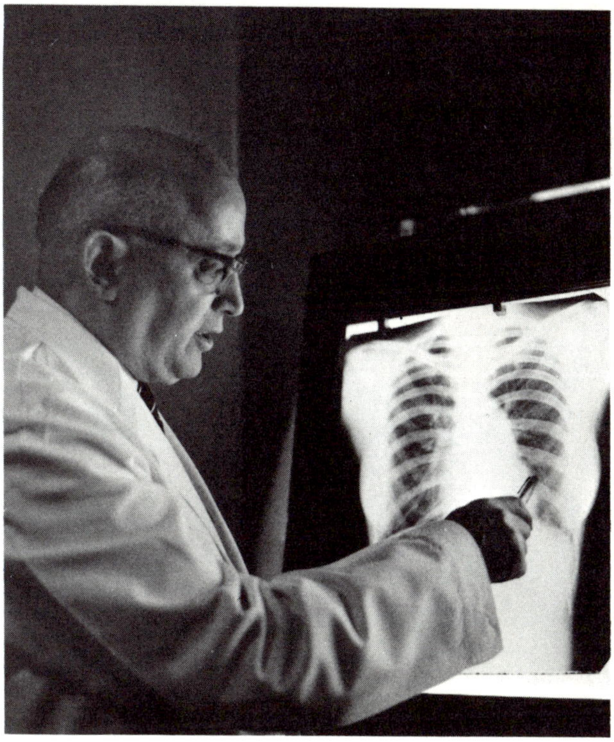

A first step in the treatment of allergic asthma is a complete physical examination. Skin tests are conducted for patient's reaction to possible allergens. A minute amount of allergenic extract is injected into the skin. A positive reaction consists of a wheal, indicating the patient is allergic to that particular allergen. The nose and throat are examined and x-rays are taken of the sinuses and lungs. Future therapy is determined by the physician after history, physical examination, skin tests, nose and throat examination, and x-rays are completed.

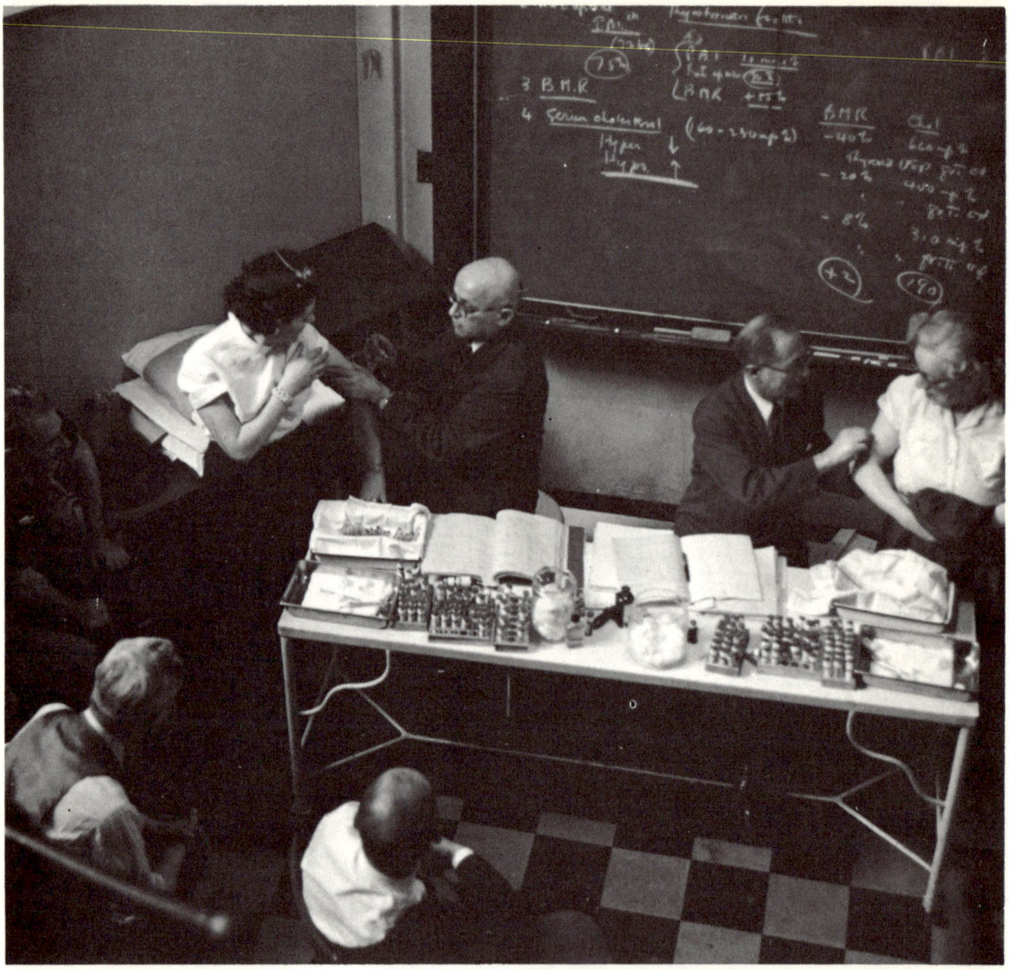

At an allergy clinic patients receive injections of allergens to which they are sensitive in order to build up a tolerance to these substances. Dosages are increased at each weekly visit.

Vacuum cleaner dust, a common source of trouble for asthmatics, is being transferred *(right)* into a pan for extraction by a medical technician. Allergenic extracts to be used in testing and treatment will be prepared from this dust.

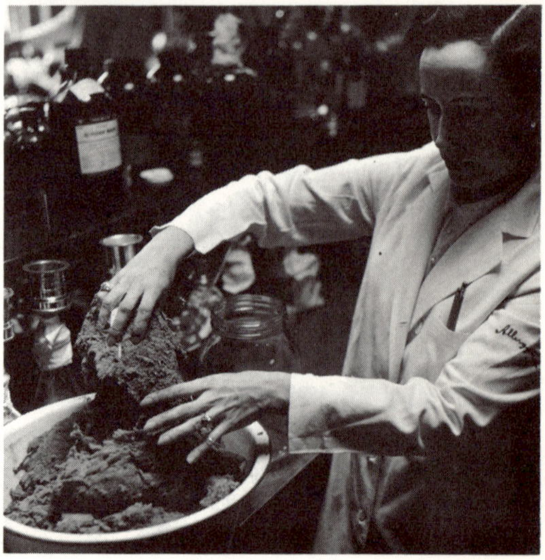

About half the incidence of asthma is due to allergy-irritation of the bronchi by specific allergens breathed into the respiratory system. The balance of the asthma cases are brought on by specific infections in the bronchi. The allergens causing allergic asthma are the same as those which are responsible for hay fever, and include pollens, organic dust, house dust, feathers, and so forth. The reason that these allergens should affect the lungs and bronchi rather than the nasal passages as in hay fever is not known. Allergic asthma begins most often between the ages of twenty and forty, while asthma caused by infection tends to occur in older people, although it can occur at any age. The disorder is generally equally divided between men and women. In both types of asthma the mucous membrane of the bronchial tubes swells and the air passages are partially closed.

A sudden asthma attack is apt to be more frightening than it is dangerous. The affected person finds himself suddenly unable to fill his lungs, and then when he has struggled to gasp in a partial breath is unable to expel it. The person in an asthma attack may bend over slightly to aid his breathing efforts. In prolonged or especially severe attacks, there may be evidence of *cyanosis*—the blueness of the skin that indicates that the blood had been unable to pick up sufficient oxygen from the lungs. Attacks rarely last for more than a few hours and are often of much shorter duration, although often the condition will persist for a much longer time in milder form with a slight wheezing noise evident in the sufferer's breathing.

The tests for the antigen involved in allergic asthma are very similar to those performed in the search for the causative factor in hay fever. The timing of attacks is carefully charted to ascertain whether they occurred after any one action of the sufferer, such as visiting in the area of a dust-producing factory, or after eating a particular food. Often the antigen is found simply by this method. If it is not, skin tests of possible culprits are made and the subsequent treatment will involve avoidance of the particular substance or substances responsible.

Treatment of the acute serious attack is usually by injection of *epinephrine,* or *adrenalin.* This is always prescribed and almost always administered by a doctor. For those people subject to frequent, comparatively mild attacks, the physician will often prescribe the inhalation of adrenalin by use of a nebulizer or atomizer. Sometimes, drugs like *ephedrine* are taken internally to produce relief. *Antihistamines, cortisone* and *ACTH* are also used to some advantage.

Often, people who suffer from allergic asthmatic attacks will outgrow the tendency—however, this is by no means always the case. The asthmatic must learn to avoid the cause of his condition and to control it when it appears. *See also* AL-

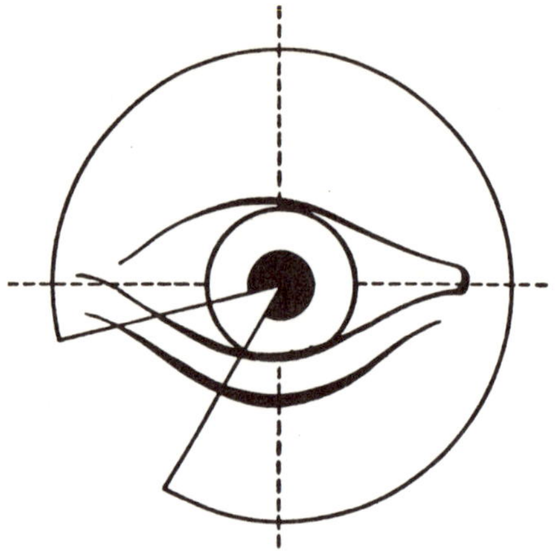

Astigmatism—A chart of the mechanism of astigmatism showing the four planes of distortion because of curving of the eyeball.

LERGY; BRONCHITIS; HAY FEVER. *See* MEDIGRAPHS pages 439, 1259, 1273, 1965, 2087.

► Allergy and Clinical Immunology, *Treatment of Asthma,* 137.

ASTIGMATISM, faulty vision which results from irregularity in the curvature of one or more refractive surfaces of the eye. When the eye is at rest, and parallel rays are focused exactly on the *retina* (the seeing tissue at the back of the eye), vision is said to be normal. The human eye is farsighted when the rays of light focus in back of the retina, or nearsighted when the rays of light focus before the retina. When parallel rays of light coming into the eye are focused at different meridians, or angles, the eye has astigmatism. Astigmatism is usually due to a change in the curvature of the *cornea,* or outside membrane of the eye, sometimes with some shortening or lengthening of the diameter of the whole eyeball.

Occasionally astigmatism is caused by defects in the curvature of the lens of the eye. The exact origin of these anatomic differences is not known beyond the fact that the shape of the eyeball varies in different people so that a tendency for astigmatism appears in members of the same family. The shape of the eyeball itself is inherited. However, injury, inflammation, or operative procedure on the cornea of the eye have been known to change the curves and produce astigmatism. Apparently, too, pressure on the eyelids may distort the eyeball and cause astigmatism.

Probably every eye has some astigmatism. However, many people do not have it enough to warrant special attention. In other cases, astigmatism causes blurred vision which necessitates corrective eyeglasses to properly focus the rays of light on the retina. When the degree of astigmatism is great, the acuteness of vision diminishes for both distant and near objects.

The specialist who examines the eyes is likely to suspect astigmatism when the eye cannot see the line of letters numbered 20 at a twenty-foot distance with the aid of spherical lenses. A simple test is made with the astigmatic dial, a clock with lines radiating to each of the hours. If the person is unable to see all of the rays with equal clarity, astigmatism is responsible. The lines that are seen more distinctly and the lines seen least distinctly indicate the principal meridians. By the amount of blurring, the eye specialist can determine the areas in which curvature of the lens needs correction. *See also* EYE.

ATABRINE, known as *quinacrine hydrochloride* in the U. S. Pharmacopoeia, was developed during World War II as a substitute for *quinine,* used in the treatment of malaria. *See also* QUININE; ANTI-MALARIAL DRUGS.

ATAXIA, disorganization of muscular coordination so that movement can be controlled only partially. It is a symptom rather than a malady.

One of the best known ataxias is *St. Vitus' dance,* in which an abnormal nervous system, perhaps as a result of streptococcus infection, causes constant sharp twitching of various parts of the body. Another ataxia is *multiple sclerosis,* in which sections of the nervous system degenerate and form scar tissue, which causes partial paralysis, among other symptoms.

Parkinson's disease, also known as *shaking palsy* and *paralysis agitans,* manifests itself in trembling and loss of power in the muscles. *Locomotor ataxia,* characterized especially by muscular disorganization and disordered sensation, is the result of infection of the spinal cord by *syphilis.* Several other special ataxias are known, including that which affects children suffering from *cerebral palsy.*

Any symptoms, such as loss of control over certain muscular movements or unusual involuntary movements in the muscles, should receive the immediate attention of a doctor, preferably a neurologist, a specialist in nervous disorders. Although the condition may be temporary, a major disturbance of the nervous system is a serious condition. The doctor will know which ataxia is involved, and often, if the condition is a degenerative one, he can take measures to retard or even stop its advance.

Some particular ataxias are hereditary and make repeated appearances in the same family. Such ataxias, the result of a localized developmental failure in some part of the nervous system, may affect not only muscular movement but also the sense of sight, touch, hearing, taste, or smell.

In cases of cerebral palsy, lack of coordination, most commonly associated with generalized muscle weakness, is notable. Treatment consists of muscle-strengthening and coordination exercises. *See also* CEREBRAL PALSY; LOCOMOTOR ATAXIA; MULTIPLE SCLEROSIS; PARALYSIS AGITANS.

ATELECTASIS, complete expansion or partial collapse of the lung. It may be present at birth or result from disease of the lungs or bronchi. It is a condition in which the air is lost from the small alveoli, or air chambers, in the lungs, giving the lung a contracted, solid appearance when viewed with the x-ray. *See also* LUNGS.

ATHLETE'S FOOT (*tinea pedis*), a ringworm infection or *dermatophytosis* of the feet, is a superficial fungus disorder. It is not restricted to athletes, but is found in all age groups and in both sexes, although it occurs more frequently in men. Usually the infection occurs where skin surfaces meet, such as between the toes, and, more rarely, the fingers, groin, and under the arms. Tight, ill-fitting shoes, heavy nonporous socks, sweaty feet, the use of public showers and locker rooms with damp floors all contribute to the spread of the infection. Acute cases usually begin in hot weather or in moist tropical climates, although chronic and sporadic cases may occur at any season of the year. When the skin tissues are softened by perspiration or moisture, the surface acidity of the skin is decreased and more susceptible to infection.

There are three types of athlete's foot, determined by the kind of fungus which attacks the skin, and the mannei in which the tissues react. In the *acute*, weeping, highly inflamed stage, little blisters appear singly or in patches between the fourth and big toe, with scaling, cracking, and oozing of the skin, which may spread to the undersurface and sole of the foot. The more *chronic* form, *intertriginous*, begins with a crack in the skin between the fourth and big toes, and formation of loosely clinging dead skin beneath which can be seen red shiny raw tissue. The *dry scaly* form, *hyperkeratotic,* is a pronounced thickening of the skin. All three types may spread to cover a portion or the entire surface of the sole.

Cracked, peeling, or sodden skin, or blisters and scaling of the feet may not always be due to a fungus infection. These may be due to *contact dermatitis,* a reaction of the skin to shoe dye, to certain chemicals in rayon or nylon stockings, or merely the result of constant friction from ill-fitting shoes or stockings. This condition requires different treatment from athlete's foot.

Treatment of athlete's foot depends upon the type of infection present. Do not use any advertised remedy indiscriminately. If the condition is the result of allergic sensitivity, these remedies may not only be ineffectual but may actually lead to more serious secondary infections. The diagnosis should be made by a physician, who may take a scraping of the infected area for microscopic examination and cultures of the suspected material. Patch tests are also made in some cases to determine whether or not a sensitivity to dyes or chemicals in the footwear causes the condition.

The fungi responsible for athlete's foot are normally found in the dead, superficial layers of the skin, so that a continuous possibility of reinfection exists. When the skin is moist and warm for a long period of time, the fungi again become active. Contact of the bare feet with organisms picked up around swimming pools, shower baths, or locker rooms may also stimulate growth of fungi. The fungi produce allergens which cause an eruption on the feet. The eruption itself may not be severe, but the allergens enter the blood stream and are carried to other parts of the body; people sensitive to the fungi or their products then develop secondary eruptions on the hands or elsewhere. This type of eruption, known as *dermatophytid* or "id" eruption, usually disappears after the primary infection is treated.

A universal method of controlling athlete's foot is not known. However, the toes must be kept clean and dry at all times, and friction in that area avoided. Dusting the feet freely with foot powder each day and after baths helps keep the area dry. Sandals or perforated shoes and highly absorbent cotton socks permit the evaporation of sweat, and help absorb moisture between the toes Small cotton wads inserted between the toes help to absorb perspiration. Paper slippers or bath clogs worn in public bathing places lessen contact of bare feet with the fungi. These simple precautions are effective in controlling athlete's foot and in eradicating milder cases.

In acute cases with reddened, blistering, weeping skin, the use of wet compresses once or twice a day, with mildly astringent agents such as *saturated boric acid* or *Burow's solution* diluted in twenty parts of water, is beneficial. When the acute inflammation subsides, a *calamine lotion* may be applied. In the acute stage, the use of antiseptics or advertised remedies may be harmful. Some leading dermatologists believe that once the acute phase has subsided under suitable treatment, prolonged therapy with a simple mild foot powder is usually enough to control the symptoms of athlete's foot. They all caution that indiscriminate self-treatment of the infection with prepared ointments may lead to more serious inflammation.

For the chronic stages, the treatment usually suggested is to soak the feet in a diluted solution of *potassium permanganate* for half an hour daily, and then to remove the crusts, scales, and dead skin. A *sodium propionate ointment* may be applied overnight and removed the following morning, and the feet dusted with a 15 per cent *calcium propionate talcum powder*. *See also* CONTACT DERMATITIS; SKIN; RINGWORM. *See* MEDIGRAPH page 1149.

ATOMIC BOMB. One of the chief effects of the atomic bomb is to destroy the bone marrow. This results in failure to develop cells so that a condition called *aplastic anemia* may develop. As a result of the loss of white blood cells, *agranulocytosis* or disappearance of white blood cells follows like the loss of the thrombocytes in *thrombocytopenia. Leukemia* was found far more frequently among persons living in areas where atomic bombing had occurred. The observations made at Hiroshima and Nagasaki established facts about what happens when a city is subjected to the explosion of an atomic bomb. According to a group of experts who have had extensive experience in this field, it can be assumed that the amount of induced radioactivity or contamination with radioactivity in the vicinity of the explosion is negligible. Teams of medical workers can enter the area immediately.

The first problem is the treatment of external injuries resulting from radiation burns, the effects of blast, and penetrating injuries. The authorities say that a third of the population of the bombed city will be killed outright or will die in days to weeks no matter how soon they are given medical care. The next third of the population will live if they get medical care quickly and if it is adequate. The remaining third can survive without medical aid unless they happen to be subjected to an epidemic or the destructive results of the disruption of transportation, sewage system, water supplies, and similar facilities.

Experience with the burns resulting from atomic bombs indicates that most of these patients ought to be taken immediately to a hospital, where they are given the modern treatment of burns. These burns are manifested by swelling, redness, and the formation of blisters. The burns resulting from irradiation are much more serious.

What treatment can be given to people who have been exposed to the effects of the atomic bomb? All of the blood disturbances that have been mentioned are best treated with daily transfusions of whole blood. Large doses of the antibiotic drugs like penicillin are given to control the infections. When there is a severe destruction of the white blood cells, these are needed particularly because the body has no defense against infection. The physician must treat the severe inflammations of the bowels, the accumulation of water in the body, and the diarrheas. Frequently it becomes necessary to give nourishment by injection. Since the patients are apprehensive, frightened, and mentally disturbed, sedatives are needed to restore their balance. In radiation burns the pain persists for days and drugs may be needed to control this pain.

We are just beginning to understand the serious problems associated with atomic warfare. What disturbs the experts particularly is the possibility that water and food supplies could be contaminated by radioactive isotopes which would themselves be taken into the body and which localize in bone and destroy human beings. Whole cities could be made uninhabitable and water supplies could be hopelessly contaminated by this method. Protection of communities against atomic bombs constitutes one of the major problems of modern medicine. *See also* RADIATION SICKNESS; LEUKEMIA; RED BLOOD CELLS, DISEASES OF; WHITE BLOOD CELLS, DISEASES OF; AGRANULOCYTOSIS; FALLOUT PROTECTION; ATOMIC ENERGY IN MEDICINE; RADIATION; RADIOACTIVITY.

ATOMIC ENERGY IN MEDICINE. Many years of experience with radium and x-ray apparatus have taught doctors much about radiation—the good that it can do and also the constant menace of harm. Radiation in minute amounts occurs almost everywhere. The earth is constantly showered with radiation from cosmic rays and traces of such radiation are found in soil and water. The means of detecting radiation include the use of photographic film and various instruments such as the Geiger counter. By the use of these devices workers are assured of safety in various industries in which radiation may be a hazard.

Radiation may damage the protoplasm which constitutes the basic materials of the cells of the body. It may affect enzymes and changes may occur in the genes and chromosomes of the cells which determine heredity. A heavy dose of radiation may destroy a cell but smaller doses may so damage the cells that children are born with congenital malformations.

Radiation is measured in *roentgens,* after the man who discovered the x-ray. This is an arbitrary term of measurement. A human being is killed with a dose of roentgens ranging from 200 to 600, or averaging about 400, that may reach the body at one time.

Radiation may reach the body from x-ray apparatus or from inhaling or swallowing radioactive material. People may be sheltered against radiation by shields such as

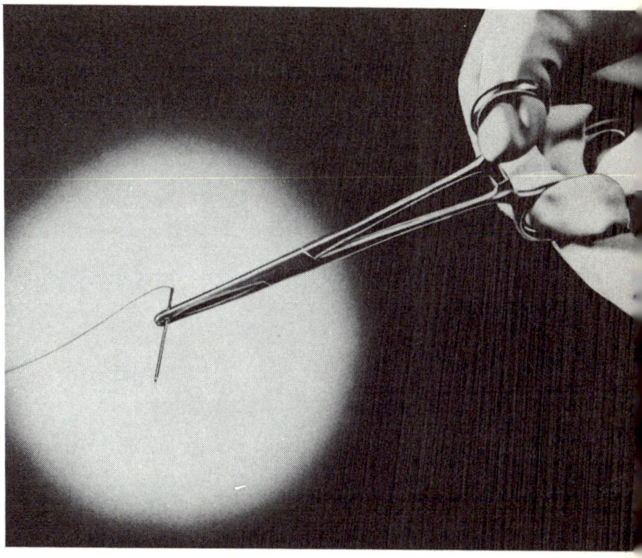

Radioactive Cobalt—After cobalt has been irradiated in an atomic reactor, it becomes strongly radioactive itself. Because radioactive cobalt is much cheaper, it has almost completely replaced radium in the treatment of cancer. A Cobalt-60 needle is pictured here. It is used to place the radiation next to cancerous tissue. Note that the needle is handled by a long forceps in order to give the physician the additional protection of distance from the needle.

lead, or by walls of brick or cement. In certain industries special installations are necessary to protect workers from radioactive dust. The workers wear photographic film badges which record how much radiation is received. The film becomes dark when radiation reaches it. In these industries the film badges are examined and checked each week. Physicians also examine the workers regularly as a precautionary measure.

Through research, which has gone on since *radioactive isotopes* were first developed, information has accrued as to how such materials may

ATOMIC ENERGY IN MEDICINE

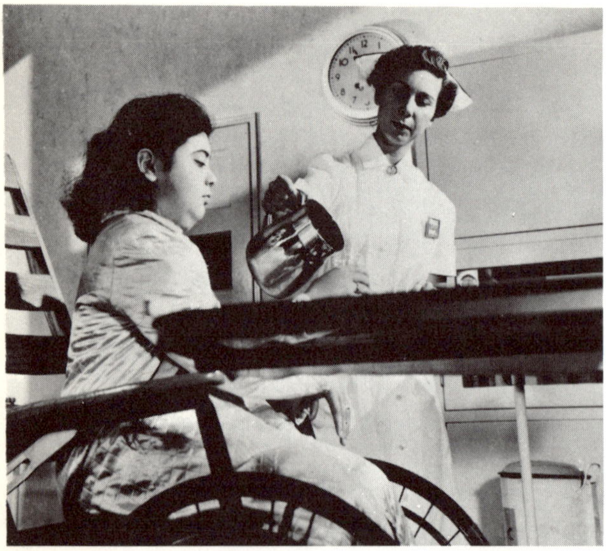

Atomic Energy in Medicine—A thyroid cancer patient is being helped by a nurse after taking a tasteless solution of *radioactive iodine*. Iodine is taken up by the thyroid tissue, both normal and cancerous. The cancerous tissue is sensitive to the radioactive bombardment and is destroyed by it. The normal tissue is not affected.

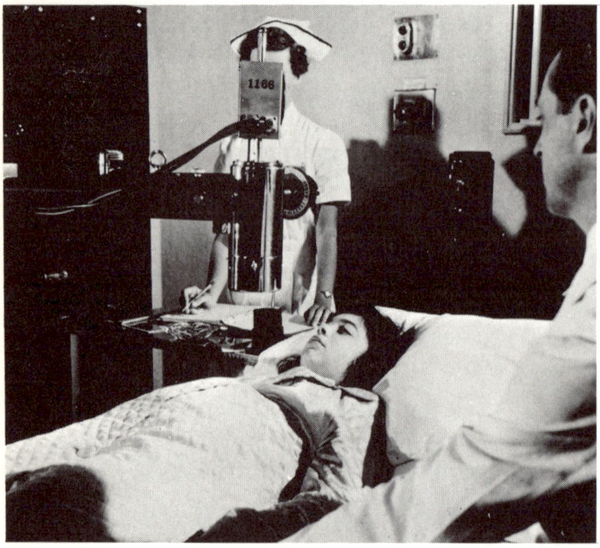

Atomic Energy in Medicine—The radioactive iodine is traced in the patient by a radiation-counting instrument. By determining the location of the radiation and measuring the strength, the effectiveness of treatment can be verified.

be used for benefiting human health. In the human body radioisotopes, which are elements made radioactive, have been used to trace the amounts of various substances in different parts of the body. For instance, *radiosodium* can be injected into the blood and the speed of the circulation determined at various points of the body. This technique may help in determining whether blood vessels are still open or whether they are obstructed by clots or hardening of the arteries. Many substances such as *digitalis, colchicine, iodine,* and *nicotine* in the form of tobacco have been made radioactive and then traced in various organs of the body. In this way medical scientists have learned how various radioisotopes act in the human body.

Radioactive iodine has been especially important to medicine. When iodine is taken into the body it goes for the most part to the thyroid gland. By measuring the amount and the rate of uptake of iodine in the thyroid gland, the doctor can determine how well this gland is doing its work. Thus the conventional basal metabolism test is in many places being replaced by the radioactive iodine test. Moreover, the iodine can take the radioactivity with it to the thyroid gland and in this way it has been used to treat *cancer of the thyroid*.

Other radioisotopes have also been used in treating disease. *Radiophosphorus* has been used to lessen the number of red blood cells in

ATOMIC ENERGY IN MEDICINE

the condition called *polycythemia* and it also has shown beneficial results in chronic cases of *leukemia.* Radioactive materials have been used to help in locating tumors of the brain and also in treating other forms of cancer. *Radiogold* has been one of the isotopes used in certain cancer cases.

Radiation, besides being used to combat cancer, can also be a cause of cancer, as revealed in follow-up studies of Japanese who received excessive doses of atomic radiation when the bombing of Hiroshima took place. When radium is taken internally it tends to localize in bones and to cause *cancer of the bones.* This was revealed a number of years ago in the cases of some women who moistened with their lips brushes with a radium mixture to make watch dials visible at night.

Cobalt is an element which when placed in an atomic reactor becomes *cobalt-60.* This is a radioactive isotope which is much less expensive than radium but which can be used effectively for the treatment of cancer. Radioactive cobalt is also used to substitute for the ordinary x-ray. Another isotope used in cancer treatment is *cesium-137.* Because certain kinds of cancer cells are more sensitive to radiation than others, physicians are beginning to classify the forms of cancer which are especially susceptible to treatment with radioactive isotopes.

Strontium applicators have been found useful for the treatment of benign growths on the eye. If removed by surgery, they tend to grow back again.

As knowledge of atomic energy has increased, new facts as well as possibilities in the field of medicine are coming to notice. In Japan people have been found who were exposed to atomic energy and developed small opacities in the lenses of the eyes two to ten years after exposure to the nuclear radiation. The eye is obviously especially sensitive to such exposure. Perhaps the earliest signs of damage from radiation may be detected by examination of the eyes.

Work has been done on the development of a teletherapy unit which will use either cobalt or cesium. The cesium, a waste product of plutonium production, has only half the radiation strength of cobalt, but it has a half-life of 33 years. The cobalt must be shipped back to a reactor for recharging every two or three years. Work has also been done on a radio thulium device which, put inside the mouth, permits the taking of far better x-ray pictures of the teeth, shooting from the inside out rather than the outside in.

Still another apparatus with greater immediate possibilities is the development at Argonne Laboratory of a portable radiation device which might be used as a substitute for x-ray in military field hospitals.

From the patient's standpoint, one great advantage to be expected from all these developments is cheaper medical service. Rates for isotope

ATOMIC ENERGY IN MEDICINE

treatment should be far below x-ray and radium treatment.

The Atomic Energy Commission now has three hospitals for cancer research. One is at Oak Ridge, Tenn., another at Chicago University, the third at Brookhaven, N. Y. Patients are selected for these hospitals on the basis of whether their cases are of the type which the medical scientists are studying at the time.

The day of the atomic general hospital has not come because the science is still limited to the number and kinds of cases in which radiation treatment is effective. Medical scientists emphasize that atomic energy offers no cure-alls.

A report by the United Nations Scientific Commission on the effect of atomic radiation has brought out pertinent facts regarding its dangers to human health. A certain small proportion of cases of leukemia and bone cancer may result from natural radiation. People who are overexposed as radiologists and radium workers have a greater hazard. The Commission called attention also to the hazards of blood disorders, cataracts of the eye, and congenital malformations. Because of the protections constantly available in industries involving atomic energy, workers in these industries are found to suffer very little damage except when there is carelessness.

Investigations have shown that one-fourth to one-half of the radiation received in more highly developed countries is from medical use of x-rays, and less than one per cent is due to radioactive fallout. The benefits of x-ray far outweigh any dangers that may occur, and suitable controls have been developed to shield x-ray operators, technicians and others that receive x-ray. Unnecessary use of the x-ray, such as was carried on in shoe stores conducting x-rays of the feet, is now abolished by law in most states of the United States.

A great deal of concern has been expressed regarding the dangers of radioactive energy in foods. A British report has shown that an average diet in England contains 300 times as much radioactive material as might reach people through radioactive fallout. However, the radioactivity from diet and fallout together does not constitute a large dose. Similarly, much concern has been given to the possibility of *radiostrontium* occurring in milk due to radiation received by cows. Radiostrontium is chemically like *calcium,* which is found in large quantities in milk. Calcium is itself a protective agent against the effects of the strontium since the tissues of plants and animals prefer calcium to strontium. The highest levels of bone radiostrontium have been found in people living in areas where rice is the main food. People who get their calcium from milk and milk products accumulate lower levels of strontium in their bones.

The civilian defense organization, in anticipation that some day the United States may be exposed to the hazards of the atomic bomb, has developed much information and guidance as to what is to be done if such an eventuality occurs. A letter to the local or state civilian defense agency will bring pamphlets with full information on how to build a bomb shelter or how to utilize available facilities, including the foods, drugs and other materials that should be kept on hand in a bomb shelter. *See also* RADIATION; RADIUM; X-RAYS; RADIATION SICKNESS; ATOMIC BOMB; RADIOACTIVITY; FALLOUT PROTECTION; OCCUPATIONAL HAZARDS IN INDUSTRY; INHALING OF DANGEROUS SUBSTANCES.

ATOPIC DERMATITIS, a skin disorder, usually of psychosomatic or allergic origin, characterized by itching, dry eruptions, and the emergence of papillae, frequently in concentric zones. The term *neurodermatitis* is also applied to this disorder.

Many victims of *asthma* and *hay fever* also suffer from atopic dermatitis. It may be caused by allergic reactions to heat, cold, certain foods, chemicals, clothing or other materials. It is frequently brought about by worry and stress.

In treating atopic dermatitis, antibiotics to which the patient is not sensitive are used to control secondary infections, tranquillizing drugs are used to lower the threshold of stimulation of the nervous system, and *cortisone* and *ACTH* are used to forestall any further allergic reactions. Ointments containing *hydrocortisone* are often helpful. *Quotane* and *tronothane* are often effective in relieving itching. Some dietary modifications are usually also necessary. *See also* ALLERGY; CONTACT DERMATITIS; ECZEMA. *See* MEDIGRAPH page 55.

► Allergy and Clinical Immunology, *Infantile Eczema (Atopic Dermatitis),* 141.

ATROPHY, the normal or abnormal shrinking or an organ or cell which has previously reached mature size. Degeneration of tissue sometimes accompanies pathological atrophy.

ATROPINE. A drug obtained from the deadly nightshade plant. *See* DEADLY NIGHTSHADE POISONING.

AUDITORY NERVE, one of the sensory nerves which influence hearing and control equilibrium. *See also* EAR.

AUREOMYCIN, a yellow crystalline substance, the trade name for *chlortetracycline,* one of the newer antibiotics. *See also* ANTIBIOTICS.

AURICLE, either of the two upper chambers of the heart which receive blood from the veins. The left auricle admits the blood from the lungs and the right auricle from general circulation. An auricle is also any appendage shaped like an ear, and refers, too, to the projecting part of the external ear. *See also* BLOOD; CIRCULATORY SYSTEM; HEART.

AUSCULTATION, the detection and study of sounds produced by the lungs, heart, and other organs to help determine their physical condition. The listening device is the *stethoscope.*

AUTONOMIC NERVOUS SYSTEM. *See* SYMPATHETIC NERVOUS SYSTEM.

AUTOPSY, the examination and sometimes dissection of the body of a deceased individual for the purpose of determining the exact cause of death. *See also* BIOPSY.

AVERAGE CHILD. The term "average," which comes from mathematics, is generally used to express the same idea as "mean" or "median"—that is, middling, or halfway between the extremes. From familiarity with published statistics people have come to think of average as some sort of standard. Men, women, and children are judged by how far they meet or exceed what is considered average in looks, behavior, or intelligence. People on the street are often interviewed for the opinion of the average man.

Actually there is no average man, average woman, or average child. No individual meets average measurements in physical features, in abilities, and in social or economic status. In statistics the average has a specific meaning and usefulness, although even there it can be misleading. Sometimes it is helpful to know the average income or average age of a population or a group, the average price of commodities, the average amount of food an individual needs. When for safety reasons the number of passengers in an elevator or airplane is limited, the limit can be calculated on an average weight of 150 pounds for each adult. Requirements for children's nutrition or children's schooling are also founded on averages. But all children are not therefore expected to eat exactly the same amount of every item of food or achieve exactly the same level in every study, any more than every person gainfully employed is expected to bring home the average amount of pay every payday.

An average is a convenient tool, but it can be misleading if not used with care, especially in its application to individuals. A group of children in a playground includes many sizes because the children are of various ages. But a group of children born on the same day would also show considerable differences in height and weight. The average height of 10-year-old boys is a rough guide to how well an individual boy of 10 is growing, but any particular child may be the shortest or tallest in any group and still be developing satisfactorily. The height and weight of millions of children have been recorded in the United States and other countries, and a great deal of information has been gathered about the range of variation among normal boys and girls at different ages. A child may be considerably shorter or taller, lighter or heavier than his agemates and still be within the normal range for his age. Many other factors are considered by the doctor, besides the weight-height averages, in determining satisfactory growth.

Parents can approach other aspects of child development in the same way. Knowing that each child is unique by inheritance, they will not expect their children to be "average or better" in everything. A particular boy or girl is usually above the average in some abilities and below the average in others.

Early in the twentieth century many kinds of tests were developed to try to measure children's abilities. While in general they confirm the fact that children differ, these tests do not measure imagination, drive, emotional responsiveness, and other qualities that contribute to an individual's total personality.

To label any child average is to go counter to a great body of evidence that each child is unique. It is also unfair to the child to assume that he is limited to being average in all respects because he happens to coincide with an arbitrary mathematical measurement in one or several ways. Every child is entitled to all possible opportunities to try himself out and discover and use the various capabilities that are uniquely his own. *See also* ABILITIES; GIFTED CHILD; INTELLIGENCE.

B

BABIES, PREMATURE, babies which are born before the full term of pregnancy or which weigh less than five and a half pounds. Babies rarely survive if they weigh less than 2.2 pounds, or 1000 grams, at birth although there are records of the survival of large numbers of infants who were born weighing less than 2.2 pounds. Since these records show that such babies catch up with normal infants by the time they are six months to a year old, every possible effort is made to save their lives. Use of the incubator, breathing oxygen mixed with carbon dioxide, feeding of mothers' milk, and application of other developments of modern medical science have helped premature babies survive to become healthy children and adults.

The first step to assure survival of a premature child is to regulate the body heat. Old-fashioned incubators have been replaced by modern, electrically heated beds in which the temperature is regulated by a thermostat. Portable incubators have been developed for births taking place at home so that the baby can be put almost immediately after birth into such a device and then be taken to a hospital.

Authorities are agreed that mother's milk is the best possible food for premature babies. In most cities arrangements are now made to obtain this type for all premature infants.

The question is constantly raised as to whether babies born prematurely have the same mental capabilities as those born at the usual time. No conclusive studies have been made on this problem, but some physicians are of the opinion that premature infants born after eight months progress more slowly than full-term infants during the first year. They are somewhat slower in learning to co-ordinate during this time. It is interesting, in this connection, to realize that some of the greatest men of history were

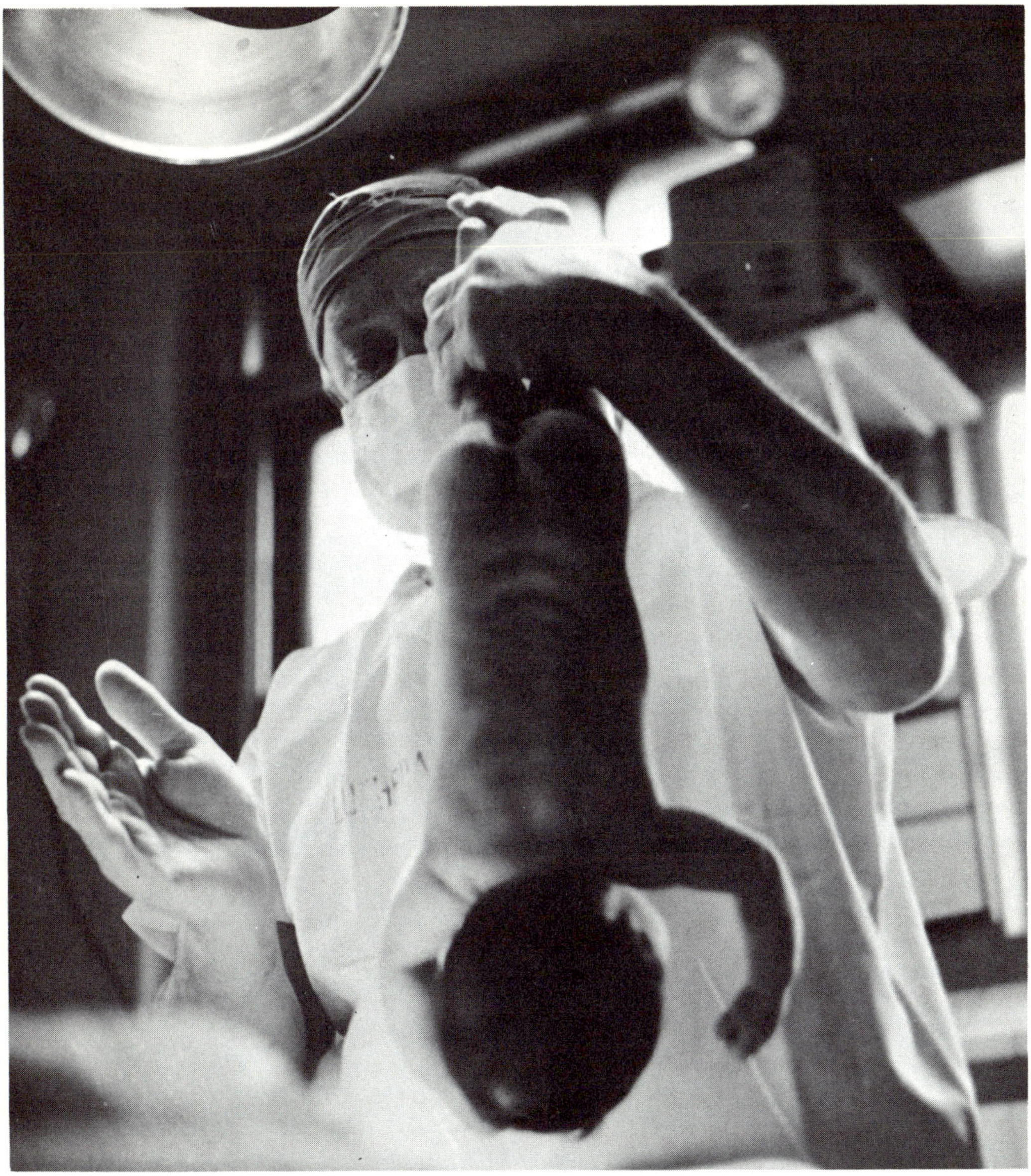

The isolette is the latest and most advanced type of incubator used in nurturing the survival of premature, anemic, or grossly underweight infants. It is a completely automatic device designed to furnish oxygen to the infant, to filter out atmospheric impurities and the carbon dioxide and moisture exhaled by the frail occupant, and to warm, cool, or humidify the air he breathes as required by his particular physical exigencies. Normally, the oxygen is administered in a 30-35 per cent concentration. However, in cases of severe respiratory disorders, oxygen is administered in a pure state. Plastic portholes in the walls of the isolette permit the entrance of the arms of a nurse or doctor for the performance of essential functions without disturbing the temperature or precise atmospheric balance. Above, a premature infant is about to be placed in the isolette. Many lives have been saved by this device.

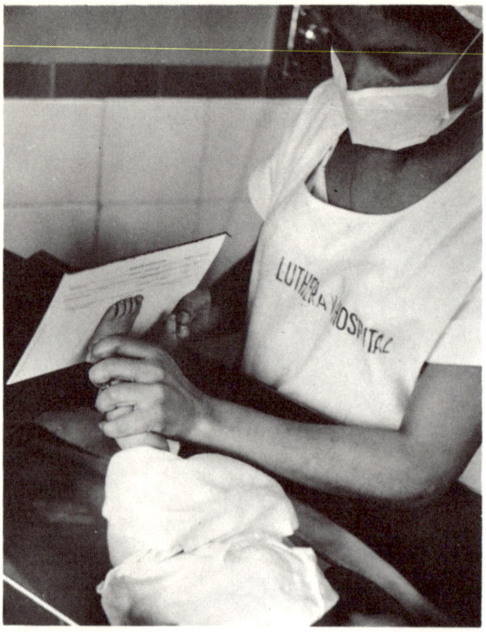

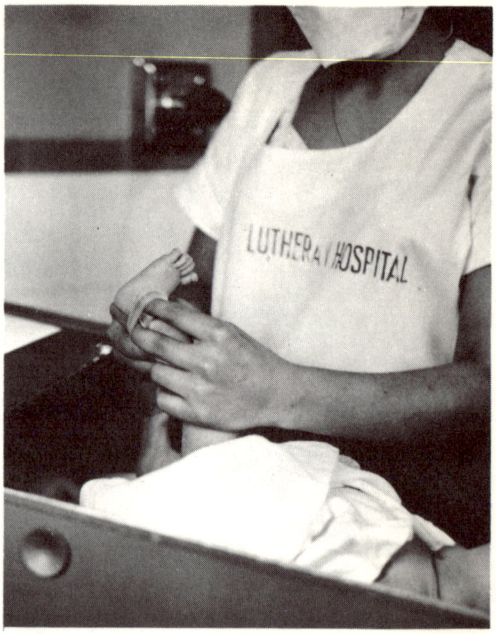

Before an infant is placed in the isolette, he must be properly designated to obviate any possible confusion as to identities. The baby is footprinted, as shown above left, and a plastic bracelet imprinted with his name is placed around his ankle, as shown above right. In the photograph below, a nurse is shown administering to the baby through the plastic portholes described on the preceding page. Note the special weighing scale designed specifically for use with the isolette.

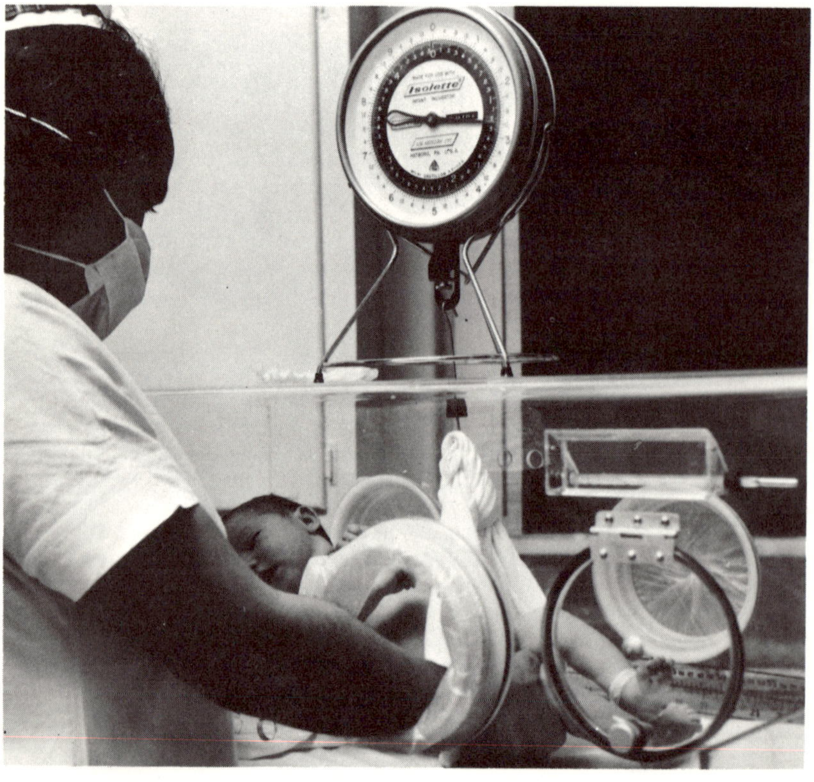

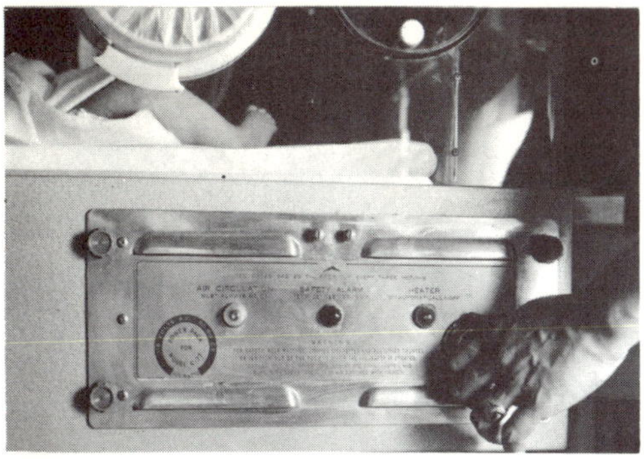

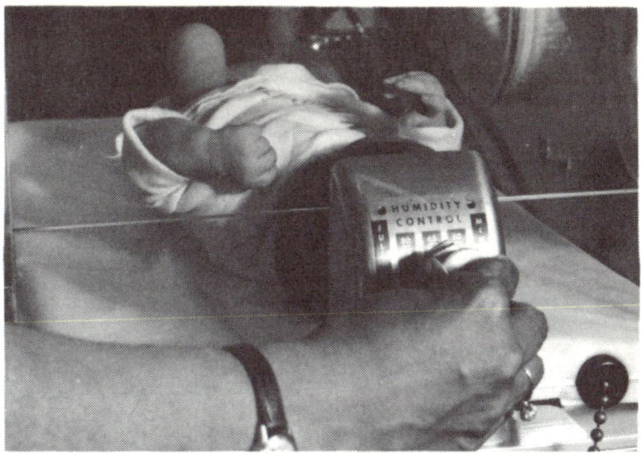

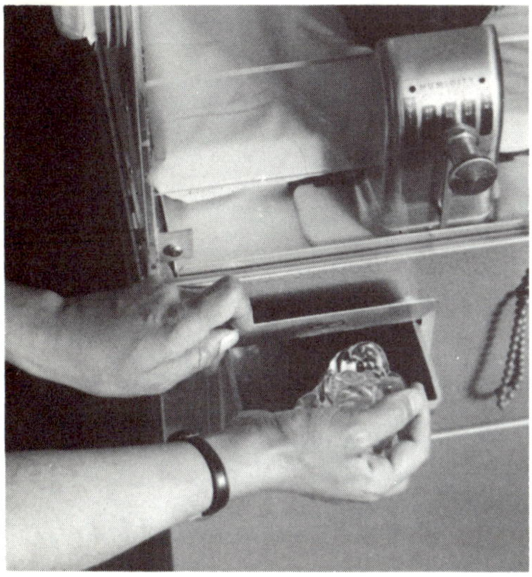

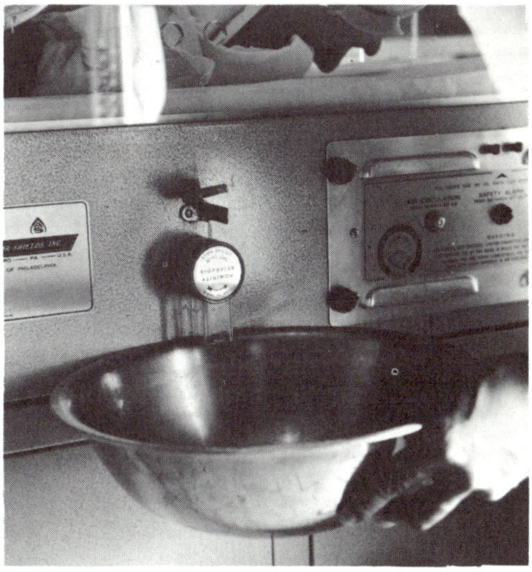

Shown above at top are some of the controls of the isolette. In the photograph at top right, the humidity control is being adjusted to conform with the baby's requirements. Directly above, at left, ice cubes frozen from distilled water are being inserted in the proper chamber. These prevent the baby from becoming overheated. At right, moisture exhaled by the infant is drained off into a pan. Below, at left, a filter for eliminating impurities from the air is shown. At right is shown the oxygen input mechanism, with printed instructions for the nurses and doctors.

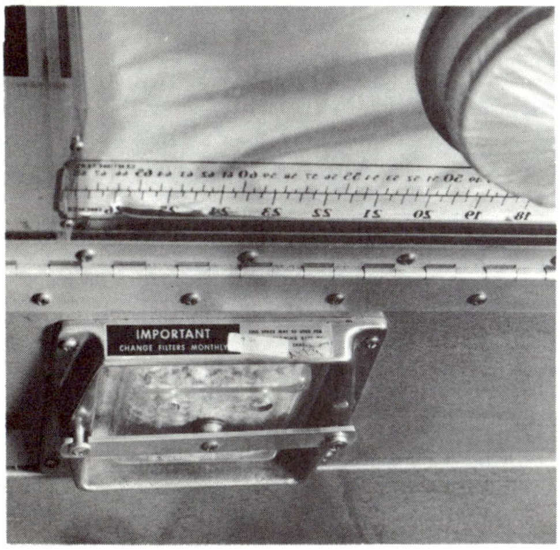

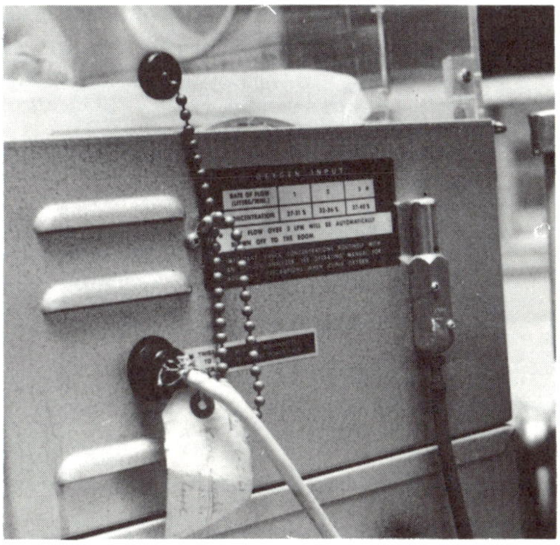

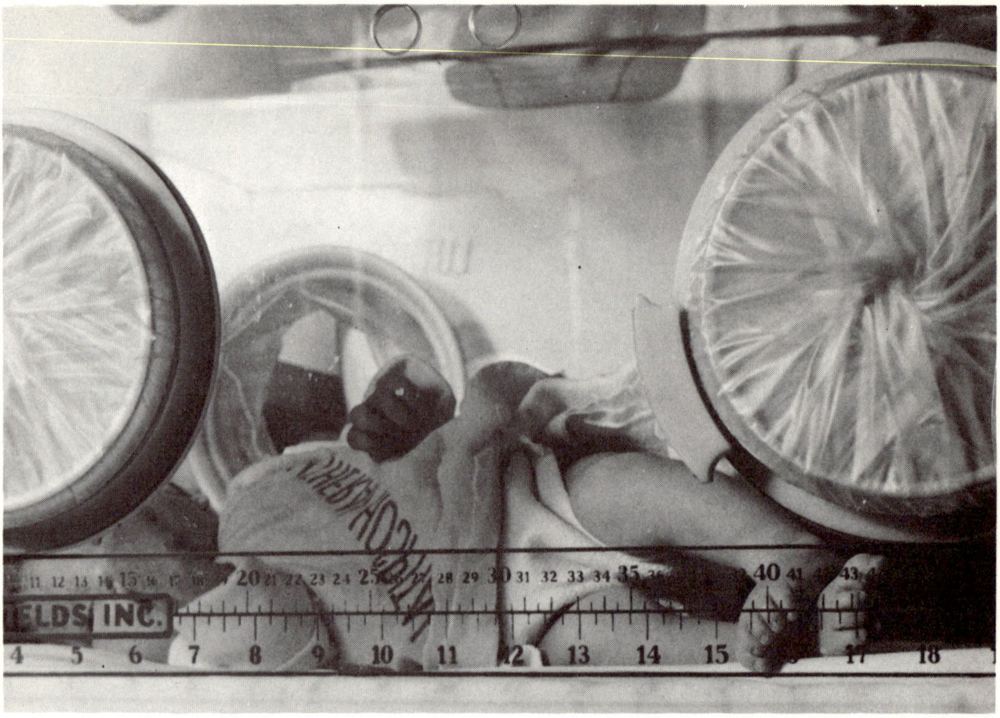

Above, the baby is measured by means of a scale printed on the plastic wall of the isolette. The nurse can be seen administering through the portholes on the opposite side. When not in use, the portholes twist shut, sealing the isolette and preventing the escape of oxygen and heat. Below, the infant, too weak to suck on a nipple, is fed with an eyedropper. Opposite, the baby, fattened up to four and a half pounds, is removed from the isolette. Careful records are kept of all cases.

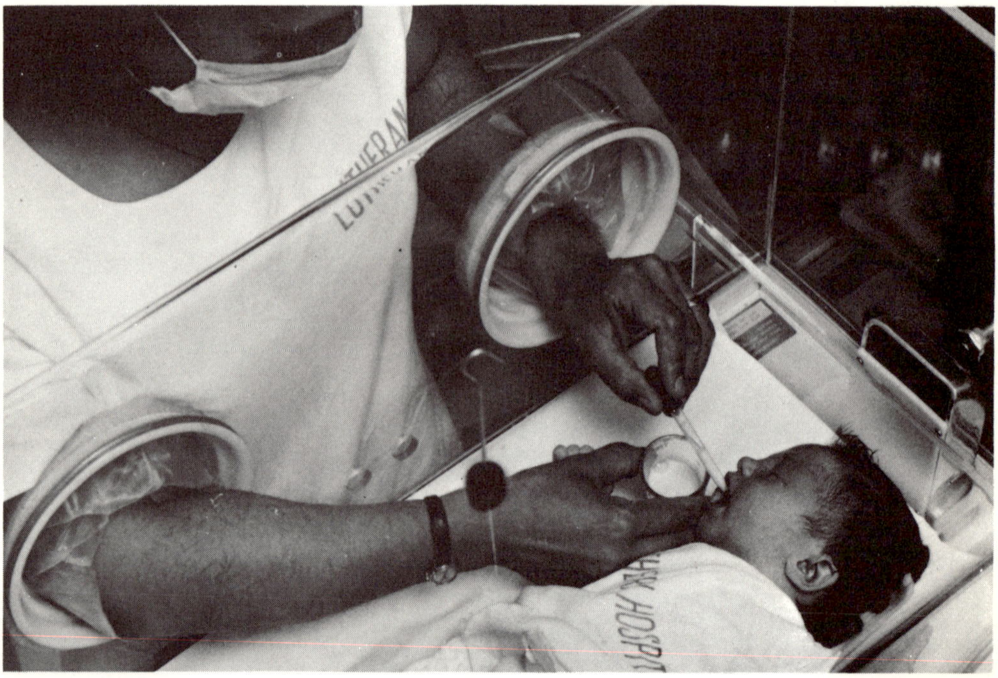

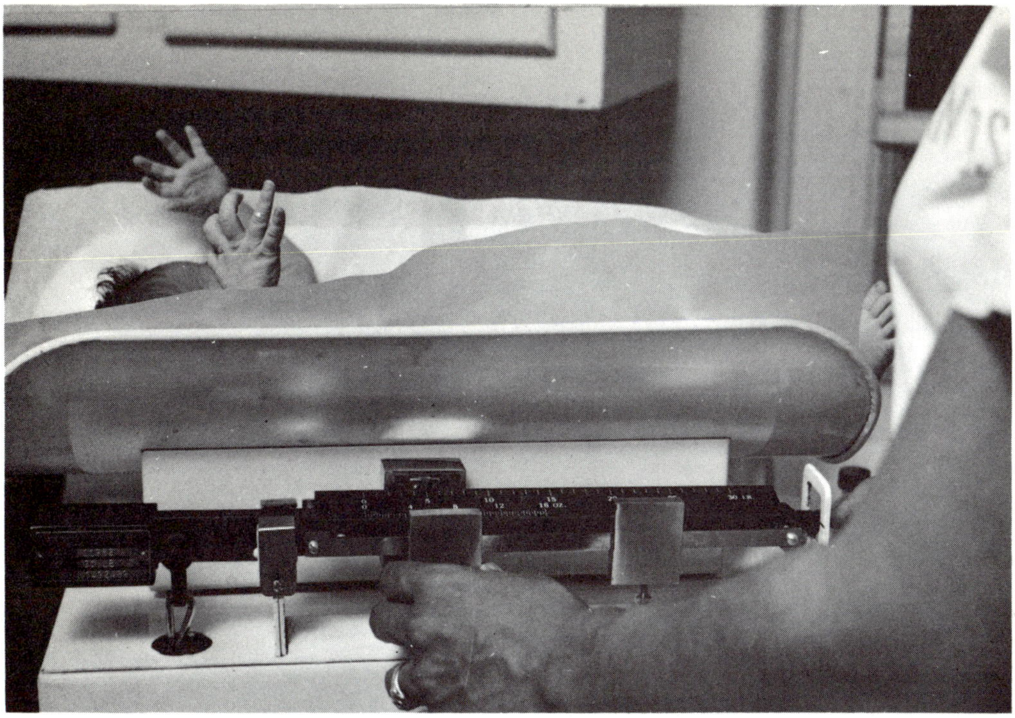

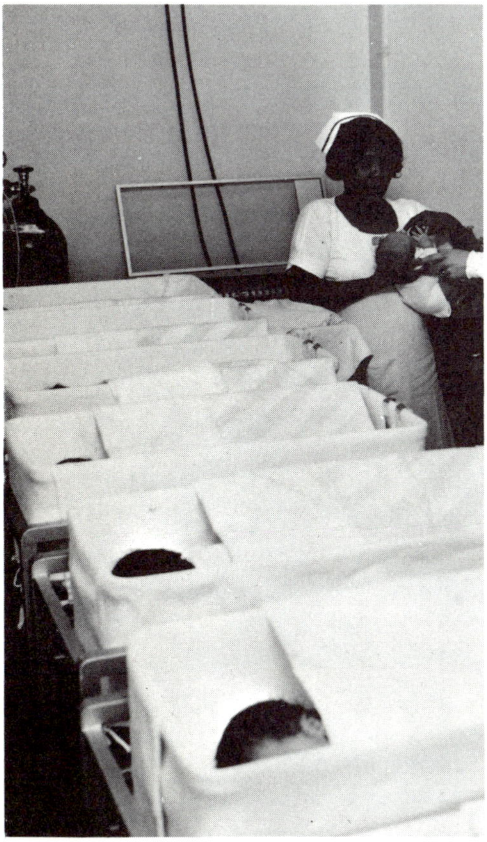

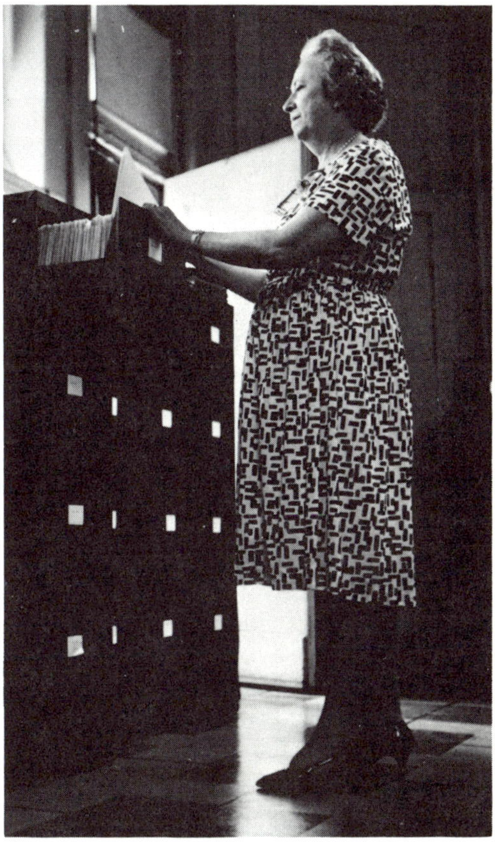

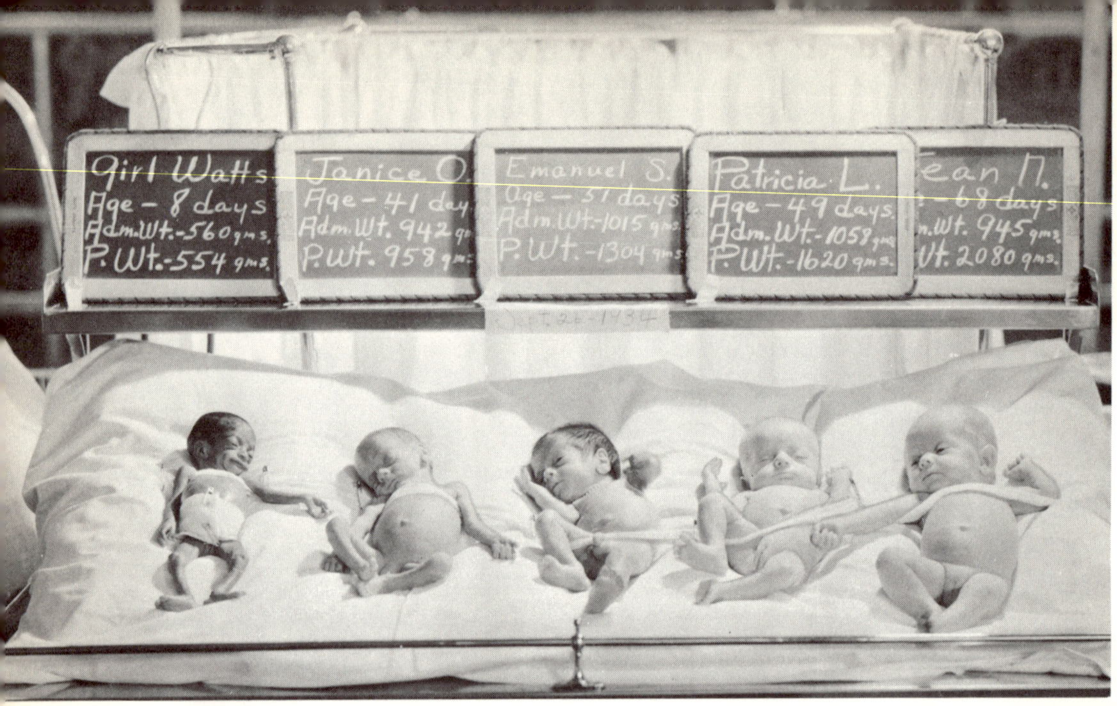

Premature Babies—Photograph of premature babies who weighed from one and a quarter to two and a half pounds at birth. Note the underdeveloped arms, legs, and hands in some of the babies. Skin is usually wrinkled and furrowed in infants who are premature.

born prematurely, including Charles Darwin, Renan, Napoleon, Isaac Newton and Voltaire. *See also* CHILD CARE; CHILDBIRTH AND PRENATAL CARE.

► Care and Feeding of the Child, *The Premature Infant,* 1801.

BABY TEETH. These are the first or primary teeth, also known as temporary or milk teeth, that come before the permanent ones. The first of the 20 baby teeth generally arrive between the fifth and eighth months, and the full set by two and a half to three years, though it's quite normal to have them earlier or later. The care of the baby's teeth actually begins before he's born—influenced by his mother's diet during pregnancy, which should insure an adequate supply of the tooth-building vitamins C and D. The reason for taking good care of the baby teeth is because they help to keep the jaw in the right shape for the development of the permanent teeth. That's why doctors usually supplement the baby's milk diet with citrus juices and some form of fish-oil. *See also* TEETH; DENTAL CARIES; DENTAL CARE; BRACES, DENTAL.

BACILLARY DYSENTERY, an acute infection of the large bowel, caused by bacilli, rod-shaped bacteria called *Shigella* (after Kiyoshi Shiga, Japanese biologist who first isolated the species). They enter the body in contaminated food or water. The symptoms of the infection include diarrhea and cramps, and it normally runs its course in about ten days and is rarely fatal.

Epidemic bacillary dysentery prevails most frequently when large groups of people are crowded together without adequate sanitation

—for example, in armies or refugee camps. World War II was the first war in which sanitation was sufficiently developed to prevent such epidemics in the field.

Sulfonamide drugs are usually effective against the invading bacteria, but if the bacilli develop resistance to sulfa, other antibiotics or drugs may be used. Prevention involves not only identification and isolation of all cases but also of carriers, persons in whose bodies the organisms live without producing in them the usual symptoms of the disease. These persons, particularly if they have an occupation such as cook or waiter, may spread the bacilli.

The symptoms of bacillary dysentery are not unlike those of *amebic dysentery, cholera, typhoid* and *paratyphoid fevers* and the *diarrhea* due to infection by *Salmonella,* another rod-shaped organism which may get into food. Special tests and examinations are therefore essential to determine the particular bacteria present in each case. *See also* AMEBIC DYSENTERY; DIARRHEA; CHOLERA; TYPHOID FEVER. *See* MEDIGRAPH page 167.

BACILLI, one of the main divisions of bacteria have a characteristic rod shape. They include a large proportion of the most significant bacteria. Bacilli of one type or another are responsible for tuberculosis, diphtheria, typhoid fever, leprosy, plague, tetanus or lockjaw, and other diseases. Bacilli are also involved in the decomposition of dead organic substances, in acid fermentation, and in various processes of wine making. *See also* BACTERIA.

BACKACHE, like headache, is a symptom rather than a disorder and, similarly, may originate from a multiplicity of causes. (*Lumbago* and *low-back pain* are words meaning no more than that the back aches.) Because of the complex structure of the human backbone, it can be subject to a great variety of disorders. Its vertical position, which enables man to walk vertically and perform tasks impossible for animals, throws a burden on the spine which most creatures are spared.

The flexibility of the backbone makes it possible to perform a number of activities which otherwise could not be done. The human spine is like a spring, curved like the letter S. The top bulge of the letter S makes up the round shoulders. The bottom of the letter S is the hollow of the back. As the human being gets older, the shoulders become stooped; the hollow in the back becomes less and then hollows the wrong way. As a man gets older, the backbone tends to form an arch instead of a spring.

The spinal column or backbone is composed of small bones between which are cushions known as discs. Inside this column is a tube which contains the spinal cord. The nerves come out in little notches between the bones. The bones are bound together by tissues called ligaments. The discs are made of cartilage.

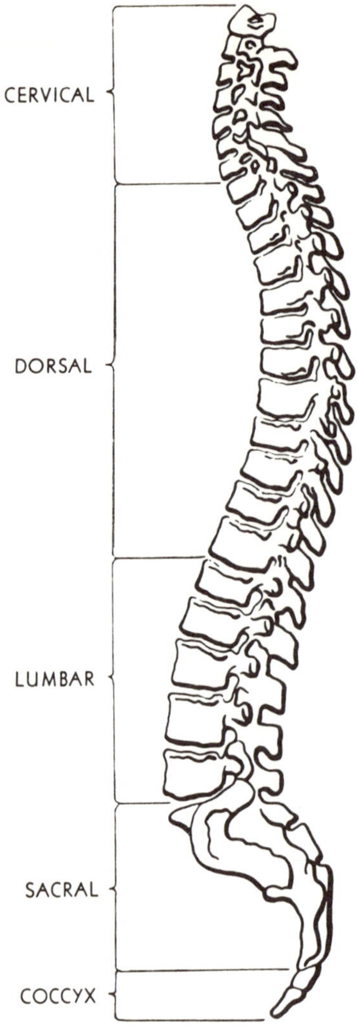

Backache—The bones of the spine (vertebral column) are classified in groups according to location. These vertebrae are movable. At the lower end of the spine, five small bones fuse to make up one large bone called the *sacrum*, or the *sacral area*, and four other bones fuse to form the *coccyx*. An intervertebral disc (not shown) lies between two movable vertebrae and acts as a cushion or shock absorber; it may be damaged or displaced under excessive strain or exaggerated motion. The spine shown above is viewed from the left side of the body, and the spiny projections seen on the right in the drawing are the tips of bones which can be felt if the finger is run either up or down the column.

Obviously an inflammation, irritation, or infection of any portion of these tissues may result in pain in the back. A sudden overstrain or a long continued strain may throw one of these many joints into a wrong position. A disease may weaken some portion so that other parts of the spine will have to carry extra strain and stress.

The back is actually one of the strongest and most important parts of the body. If it could be given the same kind of personal consideration and attention that we give regularly to our teeth, skin, and other portions of the body that are easily visible, the human body would be a more efficient working mechanism and would probably last longer without breaking down.

Back pain and back ailments may be closely related to occupations in which the spinal structure is required to absorb more stress than it can tolerate. Continued heavy lifting or prolonged standing on the feet impose unusual strains and have a perceptible effect on the body, even during a single day, and may be responsible for back pain. For example, a traffic officer who stands on hard pavement all day without rest will often lose a full inch in height between the beginning of his work and bedtime. Eight hours' rest permits the spine to spring back to its full normal length and the inch is restored.

Backache may result from infection, overstrain, disruption of some part, injury or failure to function properly in any part of the complicated spinal system. The structure of tissues of the back may have been defective from birth. Perhaps one or more of the many parts of the back have been injured or strained. Occasionally a slight difference between the length of the legs will put the whole body off balance and require abnormal effort on the part of the back to maintain correct position. Infection may attack any part of the back and is particularly troublesome when it affects the joints or the largest muscles involved. Tumorous growths may appear. Disturbances in the glandular systems and in the organs may indirectly be the source of serious back disorders. Malfunctioning of the parathyroid glands, for instance, may cause a general softening of the bones and thus be responsible for a fracture of the backbone. Diseases of the nervous system, meningitis, encephalitis, and others also produce backache.

Backache may originate with conditions which primarily affect some other part of the body, or as a by-product of surgery. Conditions as varied as stomach ulcers, gout, and disease of the gallbladder can cause back discomfort. In women, stress and strain on the tissues joining the womb to surrounding tissues, either as a consequence of pregnancy or otherwise, often produce backache. Occasionally abdominal surgery heals in such a way that scar tissue develops in a place that becomes troublesome to the back. Finally, some cases seem primarily to have a psychological basis.

In treating backache, the doctor first endeavors to establish the specific condition involved and its sources. Sometimes this is simple to do, but frequently it includes extensive tests, x-ray studies, and collection of the fullest possible medical history of the patient as well as complete information of the conditions of his work and daily activities.

Excess weight, flat feet, and other structural conditions can and should be controlled. Frequently braces which support and rest a long irritated tissue will bring relief from backache. Warmth and gradually increasing degrees of massage and exercise are also often helpful. For acute or chronic backache due to strain in the lumbo-sacral region (low-back pain), rest on a flat, rather hard surface is beneficial. Boards can be inserted between the mattress and springs to insure a non-sagging sleeping surface. As long as it does not have too much "give," the bed need not be too hard. Those who suffer from postural backache will obtain definite relief from sleeping on a flat surface and by improving their posture.

Some of the many products sold to alleviate the pain of backache do afford a temporary relief. Persistent back pains, however, are a sign of a deep disorder and the doctor should be consulted. *See also* SLIPPED DISC; SPINAL CORD. *See* MEDIGRAPH page 2177.

► Stress and Disease, *Pains in Back and Head,* 2224.

BACKBONE, another term for spine. *See* SPINE.

BACTEREMIA, blood poisoning, the presence of bacteria in the blood. When the body's natural defenses around the site of an infection have been temporarily disorganized, bacteria may enter the blood stream. Such a invasion is called *bacteremia.* Symptoms are chills, heavy sweating, or general collapse.

Bacteremia is especially severe when caused by the entrance of staphylococci into the blood stream from abscesses in the skin or bone. The migrating bacteria may set up new abscesses at distant points in the body, in the deeper tissues or in the lungs. A physician should be called promptly because time is of the essence in controlling such a situation. Infections of this type can usually be controlled with antibiotics. Before the introduction of the newer drugs, especially penicillin, fatalities were numerous. The best means for preventing bacterial invasion is to care for all wounds adequately and immediately, and to get medical attention without delay for infections of the skin, tonsils, mouth, and ears. *See also* PYEMIA; ABSCESS.

BACTERIA, one-celled organisms, scientifically classified as members of the plant world. They reproduce by fission; that is, each splits, producing two completely new organisms. Bacteria constitute one of the basic and largest classes of microorganisms. The term bacteria is preferable to the more popular name, germ, which indefinitely indicates almost any invisible, disease-causing organism. Although innumerable kinds of bacteria are known, comparatively few can live within the human body, and many of these are not harmful. However, some bacteria, known as *pathogens,* can produce such diseases as *tuberculosis, diphtheria, tetanus, typhoid fever, syphilis, gonorrhea,* and *pneumonia.*

The French scientist, Louis Pasteur, was one of the first to investigate the relationship of bacteria and other microorganisms to human and animal disease. Subsequently another scientist, Robert Koch, developed specific standards for proving that specific germs cause certain diseases. Koch's rules are: (1) the germ must be located within the body of the person or animal suffering from the disease. To verify the presence of the germ, swabs are taken of the infected area, such as the throat or ear. (2) The organisms, if grown in another body, must be able to produce a similar illness, or, if grown in a laboratory culture medium, more of the same organism capable of causing the same disease.

Bacteria are extremely sensitive to the conditions under which they live, which renders them relatively susceptible to complete control. For instance, they do not survive a high degree of heat or a lower heat sustained over a longer period, especially when moisture is associated with it. Consequently surgical instruments can be cleansed thor-

BACTERIA

Bacteria—In the laboratory, bacteria are cultivated upon nutrient substances. A doctor is shown examining test tubes in which bacteria are growing. There are many types of bacteria, most of which are not harmful. In fact, many are very essential to our living. Some bacteria, however, attack the body to produce disease. Scarlet fever, pneumonia, typhoid fever, tuberculosis, syphilis, and gonorrhea are some diseases caused by bacteria.

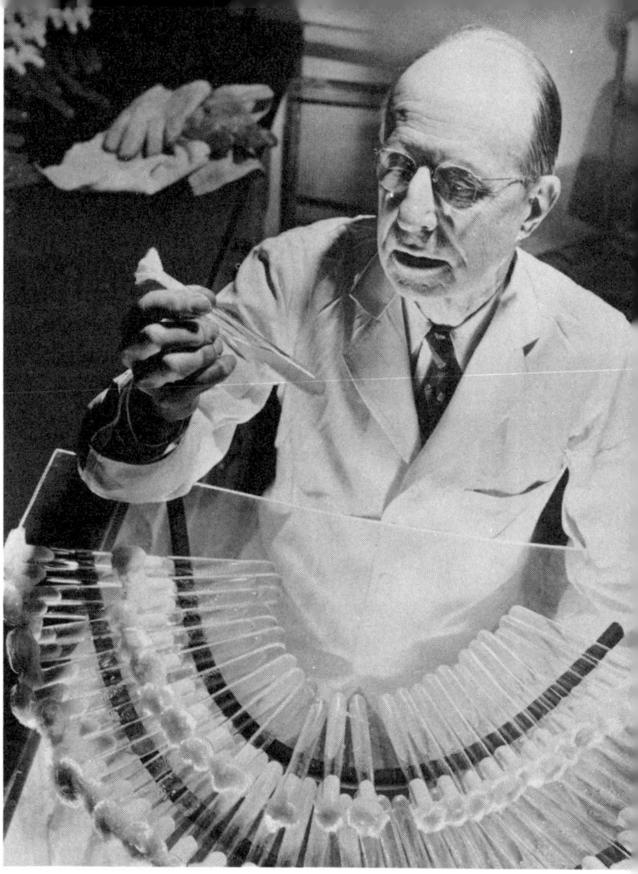

Bacteria — Microscopic pictures of bacteria which cause specific diseases. The size and shape of the bacterium are characteristics the bacteriologist looks for when helping the doctor diagnose a disease.

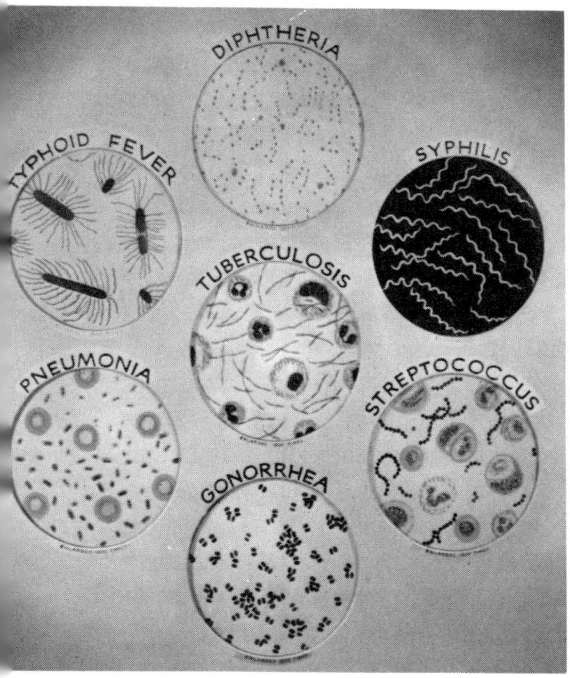

oughly of bacteria by fifteen or twenty minutes of boiling. Complete dryness, however, renders it impossible for bacteria to live, which is the reason that wound dressings are kept as dry as possible. Sunlight retards some bacteria and destroys others. Again, some germs, called *aerobic,* must have air to live; without it they die. Others, known as *anaerobic,* can live only in the absence of air.

Disease-causing, or *pathogenic,* bacteria harm the human body by the poisons or *toxins* which they produce. Some of these are excreted while others are held within the bacterial cell until it is destroyed. One of the protective measures of the body against infectious disease is the production of *antitoxins* which counteract these bacterial products. In addition the body produces other substances which prepare the bacteria for easier attack by the protective white cells of the blood, which also leads to the disintegration of the bacteria.

Bacteria usually abound wherever any moisture is present within the human environment, and protection against dangerous bacteria is a matter of selective measures rather than an attempt to avoid them entirely, which would be impossible. Eating and cooking equipment must be kept thoroughly clean for the elimination of bacteria. The hands should be washed before eating, especially after prolonged soiling or contact with anything in which dangerous bacteria are likely to live, such as human or animal wastes. Likewise bathing should be frequent.

The significance of these measures was established by a study at a midwestern university. The results proved that the effective laundering and drying of ordinary underwear cuts the bacterial count to one thousand or less per square inch, and the number rises to 400,000 per square inch in a single day's wear; that is, the numbers of bacteria present multiply 400 times, and reach 10,000,000 per square inch after underclothing is worn a week.

Since Pasteur's basic discovery in the nineteenth century, medicine has developed a formidable array of specific weapons against bacteria, in addition to cleanliness, clean water supplies, and adequate sewage systems. Antiseptics like iodine and alcohol are available to clean wounds and instruments, and immunization procedures ward off many of the worst infectious diseases, such as diphtheria, lockjaw or tetanus. In addition the antibiotic drugs, like penicillin and the sulfas, are effective against a wide range of bacterial infections. The best protection is prevention, which means maintenance of clean conditions in and about the body. *See also* BACILLI; INFECTIONS; INFECTIOUS DISEASES; IMMUNIZATION; VIRUSES; RICKETTSIAL DISEASES.

► The Skin, *Infections of the Skin, Bacterial Infections,* 2147.

BACTERIAL ENDOCARDITIS, an infection of the membranes of the heart cavities, which often attacks people who have had a previous heart disease. This condition also accounts for about 2 per cent of all organic heart disease, usually affecting young adults, although persons of every age group may have it.

Two forms of bacterial endocarditis are the *acute* and *subacute.* The acute form strikes suddenly and may cause death within a few days unless treated immediately. The subacute type comes on slowly and may also cause death within a year or so unless medical treatment is begun promptly. About 30 per cent of the cases end fatally, from various causes such as cerebral embolism and cardiac failure, in spite of treatment with the new antibiotics.

A characteristic sign is fever, especially with the acute form, although intermittent fever is usual in the chronic type. Anemia is also a symptom, as is embolism, which may disrupt circulation in acute cases, and in some instances cause nodes to appear in the skin of the fingers and toes. Fingers may also take on a clubbed appearance. Other complications include involvement of the lungs and kidney. Effective treatment of almost all cases of bacterial endocarditis consists of the use of one or more of the various antibiotics, such as penicillin or erythromycin, over varying periods of time.

For people who have heart defects and who may be susceptible to bacterial endocarditis, special care should be taken in dental or surgical treatment to prevent the possibility of its development. Such persons should be given large doses of penicillin or other antibiotics before any operation. *See also* ANEURYSM; CIRCULATORY SYSTEM. *See* MEDIGRAPHS pages 287, 1829.

► Diseases of the Heart and Circulation, *Bacterial Endocarditis,* 1291.

BACTERICIDE, any substance able to destroy bacteria.

BACTERIOPHAGE, the name applied to a virus when it infects bacteria. *See also* VIRUSES.

BACTERIOSTATIC denotes the power of stopping the growth of bacteria.

BALANTIDIASIS, or *Balantidial colitis,* an infection by a species of protozoa, unicellular bacillus, called *balantidium.* It is characterized by diarrhea and dysentery.

BALDNESS, or *alopecia,* loss or absence of hair. According to one authoritative estimate, nearly 300 million dollars a year is spent on alleged remedies and treatments for baldness. Occasionally good results seem to occur from these remedies, usually because hair, in many types of baldness, returns regardless of treatment or lack of it. This type of baldness and spontaneous regrowth often follows infectious diseases accompanied by fever, including pneumonia, typhoid, and influenza. Serious hair loss sometimes follows childbirth and surgery. In all these conditions, normal hair growth returns without help.

Bald or balding persons often wonder if there is anything that can be done to remedy their condition. The medical, and only reliable, answer at this time is that not much can be done. However, some hope for the future is held out; solution awaits the time and money needed for more thorough investigation.

Knowledge of the growth of hair in human beings has recently been broadened by delicate studies of the growth of hair using high power microscopes and other laboratory methods. Studies of the regeneration rate and the growth of human hair have brought out some interesting facts. When a hair is plucked from the scalp, approximately four and a third months pass before the hair follicle has regenerated so that it can produce a new hair. The hair grows at the rate of 0.35 millimeters per day. At least 6 months more must pass therefore before a new hair will attain its full growth. The life span of hair in the human scalp

(Continued on page 288)

the disease and its causes There are many causes of endocarditis, which is an inflammation of the lining membrane within the heart. Subacute bacterial endocarditis, the commonest form, is caused by a bacterial infection—usually the streptococcus viridans—which infects a heart valve previously damaged by rheumatic fever, or infects some congenital heart defect.

Introduced into the body via an infection, the bacteria grow and ultimately reach the heart by way of the bloodstream. Just how the bacteria establish themselves in the heart valve areas involved is still unknown. However, once established, particles composed of bacteria may break off the main clusters around the heart valves, and may be carried as infected emboli (blood clots) into the bloodstream, to all parts of the body. The damage they do depends upon their size, and the organ of the body to which they are carried. Emboli involving the blood vessels of the intestines and the brain are likely to have serious effects.

symptoms The symptoms are illustrated in the Medi-Graph. In most cases they follow an illness or some minor surgical procedure. There is no typical picture of this disease. The condition of the heart, and the extent of heart damage before the infection is apparent, will determine the effect on the patient. The course of the illness varies also, lasting from as short a time as one month to as long as two years. There was a time when this disease was without hope of cure, but now 70% of the patients respond to antibiotic therapy and survive.

complications These depend upon the part of the body involved with emboli. Congestive heart failure may appear at any time. A form of nephritis can also develop.

prevention (or lessening of impact) The underlying disease in bacterial endocarditis is often correctable. Properly diagnosed subacute bacterial endocarditis can be treated with drug therapy and managed in such a way as to minimize or avoid complications.

A patient with a rheumatic or congenital heart condition must make use of antibiotics, as recommended by his physician, whenever he has even a simple infection or is involved with any surgical procedure. He may even be put on preventive doses of antibiotics for life. A patient who has been advised that he has a correctable congenital heart condition should make use of surgery as soon as possible. The maintenance of good health and general well-being are also very important.

Subacute Bacterial Endocarditis

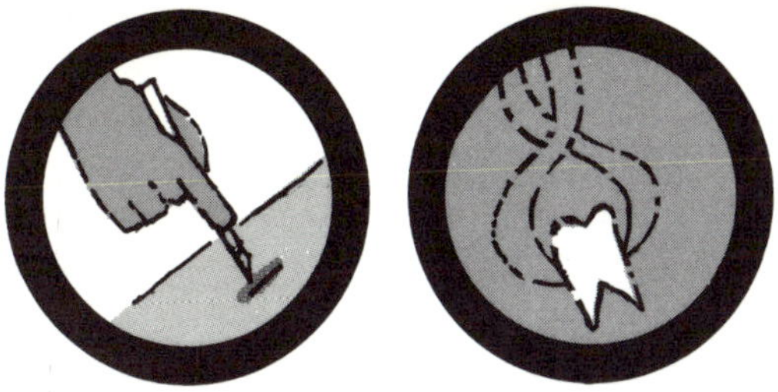

1. Bacteria enter blood stream as aftermath of minor surgery, dental extraction or other infection.

2. Bacteria reach heart and lodge in:

- **A.** heart valve—usually one previously damaged by illness such as rheumatic fever
- **B.** birth defect—such as opening in wall between 2 sides of heart

3. Clots (infected emboli) may break off growing bacteria colony and cause damage by blocking circulation or causing infection in other parts of the body.

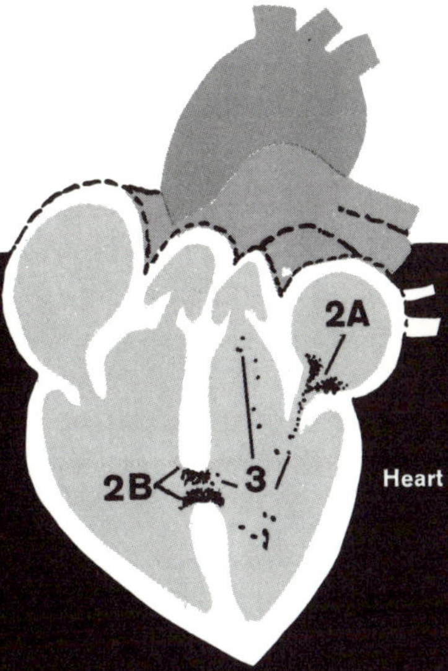

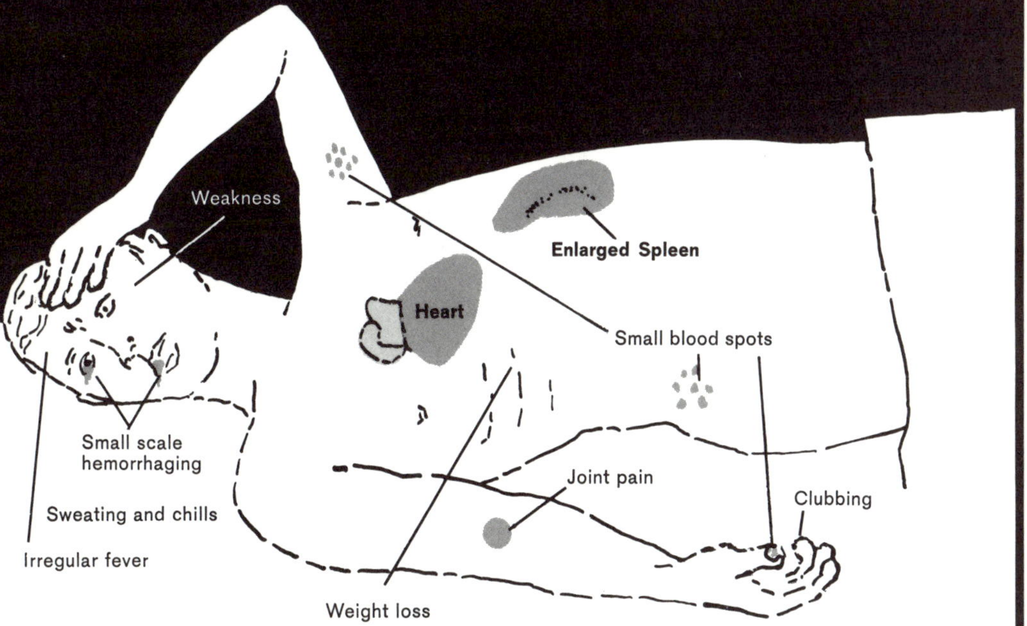

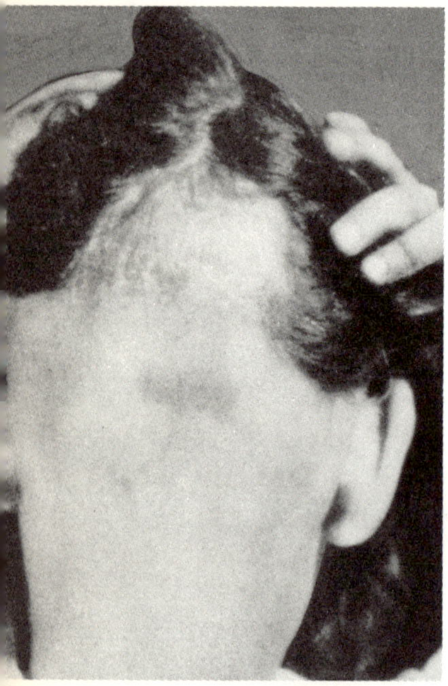

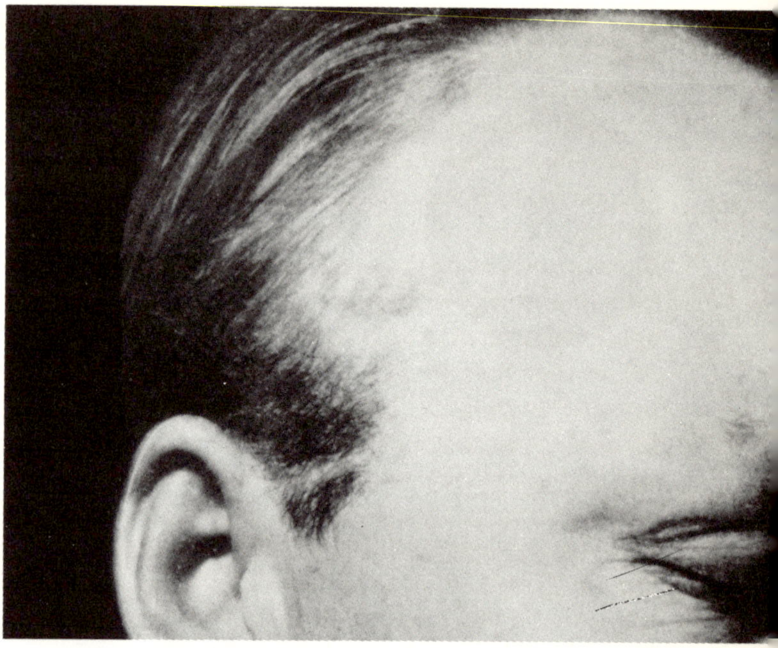

Baldness—*Alopecia areata*—a condition of baldness which occurs in patches. Bald spots may appear on any area of the body, but most often the head is involved. Loss of hair is sudden; regrowth may be slow or spontaneous and can take place without treatment. In some cases, bald spots are resistant despite all efforts to stimulate hair growth. Alopecia areata affects both sexes and the cause is unknown. Two types of area baldness are shown. The band-like type is the form frequently resistant to treatment.

is 6 months. An eyelash survives for three months and a hair of the eyebrow for 3 weeks. For many years attempts have been made to find out the exact cause of baldness scientifically called alopecia. Certain forms of baldness are definitely related to nervous shocks or stress. This condition is called *alopecia areata.* Most physicians have been convinced that the common type of baldness represents an hereditary manifestation so that men not only inherit the tendency to loss of hair at certain ages but also a certain pattern of baldness. The new studies represent the application to this subject of the newer knowledge of chemistry.

Some years ago workers in the synthetic rubber industry found that the workers who used *neoprene* in their work became temporarily bald. The fall of hair was traced subsequently to a group of chemical substances such as *chloroprene* which when applied to the skin of laboratory animals not only caused a complete loss of hair but also the disappearance of the hair follicles, a hardening of the surface of the skin and an inactivation of certain chemicals in the skin called *sulfhydryls.* The theory was then suggested that other unsaturated chemical compounds might effect similar changes. Vitamin A which is related to chloroprene was studied and it was shown that this vitamin can affect hardening of the surface of the skin and in excessive amounts may cause generalized loss of hair in both animals and humans. It did not however inactivate the sulfhydryl compounds. Among other compounds studied was one called *skualene.* A single application of skualene caused falling of the hair in rats and guinea pigs but not in mice. It did not effect hardening of the surface or cause any disappearance of the hair follicles. Hence it was suggested that skualene or related compounds in the oil glands might influence the growth of human hair. This new information does not invalidate the opinion that the glands of the body and particularly the *pituitary gland* and the *sex glands* have a definite influence on the growth of hair.

Subsequent research has shown that the *sebum* which is the main ingredient of *dandruff* contains compounds which may cause the hair to fall. Another group of investigators found that the content of the hair fat of adult women is greater than that of men.

Aristotle stated more than two thousand years ago that men and not women are usually afflicted by baldness, and today's medical science confirms this observation. Baldness seems not only to be largely restricted to males but appears also to be actually a male disorder. Some doctors believe that male sex hormones circulating in the body stimulate the sweat glands to produce a surplus of sebum which increases baldness. Attempts to counteract the effects of the male sex gland have not been successful, and neither have experiments with the female hormone *estrogen* in hair creams and lotions. Dermatologists agree that the use of estrogen in baldness may be dangerous and is thus ill-advised.

Most popular beliefs about baldness are untrue and exploited by quacks. Dry brittle hair, dandruff scales, thinning of hair in the crown and temples, tight and itching scalp actually do not cause baldness. Nor is it exacerbated by wearing hats, tight or otherwise.

Excessive falling of hair is rarely a symptom of true baldness, as has been pointed out, but more often a sign of a physical disorder which a physician should attend to. Some illness usually precedes the condition know as "patch" or "area" baldness. It may be due to any of a variety of maladies, and may clear up when the patient has recovered from the illness that caused it.

If dandruff were a cause of baldness, most people would be bald. Dandruff, the flaking of the scalp, is apparently a normal process and, in the opinion of most doctors, is not harmful to hair. Yet while the chances are great that most cases of dandruff are the simple kind, a rarer type, *seborrheic dermatitis,* cannot be disregarded. It is caused by an infection of the glands in the scalp, and produces thick scales which provoke soreness and itchi-

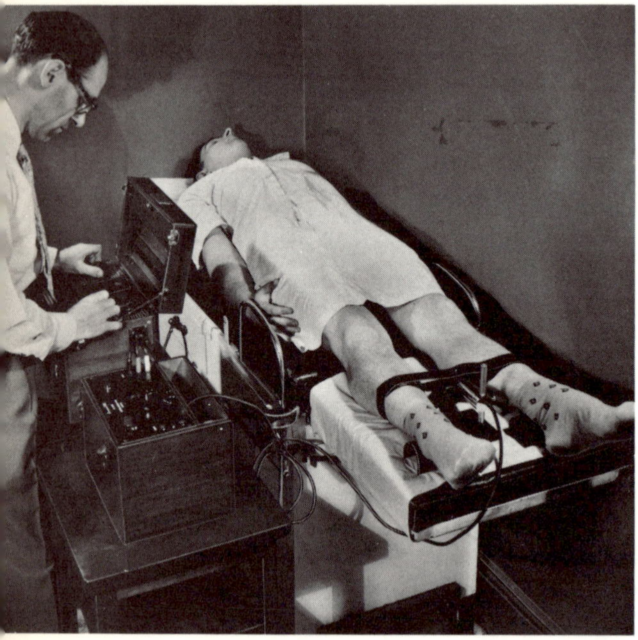

Ballistocardiography—Taking a ballistocardiogram with the Arbeit Ballistocardiograph. This apparatus records the body's recoil caused by the cardiac contraction and the ejection of blood into the aorta.

ness and may result in serious loss of hair. Research has shown that *selenium sulphide* can aid in controlling persistent seborrhea of the scalp. Two dermatologists used an ointment of one per cent of selenium sulphide but found that this might irritate the skin. When a 0.5% solution was used, few cases of irritation appeared. Studies have shown that a shampoo incorporating selenium sulphide is helpful in overcoming dandruff. A few people, however, develop reaction of the skin and even some toxic reaction when using preparations containing selenium sulphide. *See also* ALOPECIA; HAIR; SEBORRHEA.

► The Hair, *Ordinary Baldness,* 1248.

BALLISTOCARDIOGRAPHY, a technique for recording the vibration of the body that occurs when the heart contracts and throws blood into the *aorta* (the large blood vessel that carries the blood from the heart) or the recoil from this contraction. This vibration is shown as waves on a tape, and the waves vary according to the efficiency of the operation of the heart. The method is especially valuable in studying the changes that take place when the aorta is narrowed or when there is severe coronary heart disease. The ballistocardiogram has been found so sensitive that the effects on the heart of smoking a cigarette near the machine are clearly apparent.

BANDAGE, a strip of material, usually of gauze, muslin, or flannel, in rolls of varied width, used to secure dressings, to immobilize a part, to check hemorrhage and to support an injured member or to apply pressure.

BANTI'S DISEASE. *See* SPLEEN.

BARBER'S ITCH, scientifically *sycosis,* an infection of the bearded areas of the face and neck, may be caused by a fungus, *tinea barbae,* by a germ, such as *staphylococcus, sycosis barbae* or *sycosis vulgaris.*

Tinea barbae, which affects the chin and jowls and rarely the upper lip, is a severe inflammation, resulting in boggy little lumps and deep-seated sores that contain pus. At one time the infection was often spread by the use of contaminated shaving articles and towels in barber shops, but state laws which govern sanitation in barber shops have to a great extent controlled this problem. All shaving equipment must be sterilized after use, while barber's itch is being treated. Antiseptic lotions, fungicides, and ointments are helpful in reducing the inflammation. The disease is curable. If neglected, it may leave disfiguring scars; but if it is treated promptly, and the doctor's instructions followed carefully, it improves rapidly.

Sycosis barbae, sometimes caused by an infective discharge from the nose, begins with red sores around the hair follicles. The sores tend to become grouped and form pus. The condition most frequently attacks the upper lip, though it may involve the entire bearded area. The skin usually burns and is painful.

Early treatment prevents destruction of the roots of the hair and the resulting scarred and distorted skin. If the skin is inflamed, hot, saturated, boric acid dressings may be applied daily. The infected hairs are sometimes removed with a forceps until the skin seems to be healed. Soothing lotions or ointments are used at night, care being taken not to apply anything that would irritate the skin. X-ray therapy has been found beneficial in some cases. Shaving may be continued throughout the duration of the infection, but the razor should be dipped in alcohol before it is used; and a shaving cream used that does not require a brush. *See* MEDIGRAPH page 1149.

BARBITURATE POISONING. Most sleeping pills to which people become addicted are modifications of barbituric acid. Some act promptly and shortly; others act slowly and longer. People get used to depending on drugs to get them to sleep. They may take larger and larger doses. The drugs are treacherous. The person becomes stupified and confused and may take repeated doses without realizing what he is doing.

Excessive doses produce a dull sensation in the head and inability to coordinate movements. All the sensations become lessened in sensitivity including hearing, smell, taste, and the sense of touch. Nausea and vomiting may occur. Sleep may ensue leading on to stupor from which awakening is difficult. Finally the skin gets cold and clammy, the respiration is shallow and slow, the circulation gets weak and unless aroused and supported the person poisoned by barbiturates will die.

The patient poisoned by sleeping pills should be taken to a hospital where the necessary supportive measures may be applied. These include oxygen, and stimulants to the brain like *caffeine, ephedrine* and *amphetamine,* or *benzedrine.* An antidote called *picro toxin* is sometimes used as a sudden harsh stimulant but amphetamine seems to be just as certain and safer.

Some people take barbiturates habitually in small doses and get a form of chronic poisoning like a mild continuous jag. They have hallucinations, poor memory, difficulty with speech, and possible damage to the blood and circulation.

Habitual reliance on drugs is a form of psychiatric or mental disturbance which should be studied to to see if the difficulties cannot be resolved or removed. In any event the drug should be stopped and resistance cultivated, at the same time attempting to restore physical health which is damaged by all drug addictions. *See also* DRUG ADDICTION; MORPHINE AND OPIUM POISONING; BARBITURATES.

BARBITURATES, derivatives of *barbituric acid* used in medicine as hypnotic and sedative drugs. Sedatives, or hypnotic drugs, are a valuable adjunct to medicine. They can help break the cycle of insomnia in some cases, and restore the sleep pattern in others. Often they help to induce sleep when nervous and physical exhaustion has set up such a pattern of irritability that the person needs to relax for a long time. The inability to sleep can surely increase tension, making sleep exceedingly difficult. Sedation may be essential as the initial step to restful slumber.

Barbiturates are usually taken by mouth. Around barbituric acid, various pharmaceutical concerns have arranged diverse chemical groupings. Their main difference lies in absorption and elimination, onset and duration of action. In the United States, the most commonly known barbiturates are *pentobarbital,* (NEMBUTAL), *secobarbital* (SECONAL), *amobarbital* (AMYTAL), and *phenobarbital* (LUMINAL) which is the most slowly absorbed and longest acting.

Small doses of these barbiturates evoke drowsiness by depressing the functions of those parts of the brain related to mental activities. Therefore, physicians often prescribe these drugs to help patients with ulcers to relax and thus overcome contributing causes such as worry and anxiety.

Only in large doses do barbiturates have any value as *analgesics.* Some quick-acting barbiturates, such as *pentothal sodium* and *evipan sodium,* have been found effective as *anesthetics* during short operations because they rarely have any aftereffect.

In spite of newer drugs, long-acting barbiturates like phenobarbital remain a medical adjunct in *epilepsy,* in which the cerebral motor cortex is abnormally active. Barbiturates are effective because they not only produce a hypnotic effect but also slow down the activity of that segment of the brain which induces movement. Phenobarbital drugs also elicit calmness in patients in whom conditions of abnormal motor activity are produced by overactive thyroid glands.

Unfortunately barbiturates are too often subject to abuse. The physician with a patient who is psychologically disturbed endeavors to direct his treatment toward the eradication of the fundamental cause of the disturbance in preference to treating the symptoms by a long-term prescription of barbiturates. Barbiturates should serve only as a temporary bridge.

Taken frequently over a long time, and in large doses, barbiturates are harmful. As in the case of alchoholism, it is not easy to say when proper use of such drugs ends and improper use begins. The U. S. Public Health Service has stated that many people use 0.2 grams without any apparent ill effects. This equals two 1½-grain capsules, or one 3-grain "block-buster." Much more than this amount will cause various degrees of mental and physical impairment. Four times this quantity taken for only a few months will produce a dependency that may give the user withdrawal symptoms similar to those an addict goes through when the drug is removed.

The U. S. Food and Drug Administration has said of the habitual use of barbiturates, "From a purely physical viewpoint we feel that barbiturates are worse than narcotics. The habitual victim has difficulty thinking, cannot perform even simple calculations, loses the power to judge distances, becomes infantile, weeps easily and eventually has a desire for death."

According to both state and federal laws, barbiturates are not to be sold without a doctor's prescription and there cannot be any legal refilling of a prescription without specific orders from a doctor. Unfortunately the ways in which these laws are violated are numerous, and the frequent and tragic misuse of drugs which the medical profession considers useful must be curbed.

Barbiturate poisoning may be mild, moderate, or severe. Poisoning may result from a pronounced sensitivity to the drugs. Drowsiness induced by a small dose may pass into a coma after an overdose.

The symptoms of acute barbiturate poisoning resemble, to some degree, those of alcoholic intoxication. Among the numerous mental symptoms are moral deterioration, aggressive outbursts, slurring of speech, and impairment of mental activity. A reeling gait, because of uncontrolled muscular action, rapid beating of the heart, disturbed digestion and vision, and, in severe cases, exceedingly slow and shallow respiration are other signs.

Mortality, which is at present about 8 per cent in all cases of barbiturate abuse, is highest in older people and in those with a weakened physical condition. Care should be exercised not to give barbiturates to people with liver and kidney disorders, since the liver is actively involved in destroying toxins and the kidney in excreting them.

New sleeping pills, nonbarbiturates, have recently been developed. Chemists are on the threshold of developing a whole new category of hypnotic drugs safer than the powerful habit-forming barbiturates and still strong enough to induce sleep. The promising new leads have come from animal experiments with a chemical called *tertiary amyl alcohol.* This substance, known since 1890, seems to meet some of the requirements for the long-sought-for ideal hypnotic drug in that it is not habit-forming, and does not have some of the disagreeable aftereffects associated with barbiturates. Compounds of this drug produced satisfactory results. *See also* TRANQUILIZING DRUGS; POISONING; DRUG ADDICTION; SUICIDE; BARBITURATE POISONING.

► Home Care of Common Ailments, *Sedatives and Tranquilizers,* 1676.

BARIUM SULPHATE, a compound formed by *barium* and *sulphuric acid,* used as a pigment and as a filler in such products as paper and rubber. It is also invaluable in taking roentgenograms of the stomach and intestines, because, when taken by mouth, it renders those organs opaque to x-rays, and subsequently the drug passes unchanged through the gastrointestinal tract. *Barium sulphate* should be carefully distinguished from *barium sulphide* and *sulphite,* which are poisonous.

BARLOW'S DISEASE. *See* RICKETS; SCURVY; VITAMINS.

BARTHOLIN'S GLANDS. *See* VULVA.

BASAL GANGLIA, groups of nerve cells, situated internally in the brain substance. They control inherited basic emotions and deter muscles from certain movements which would occur if this area of the brain were injured.

BASAL METABOLISM. Metabolism is the conversion of food into energy in a living body. Basal metabolism is a measure of the chemical changes involved in the body at rest. The basal metabolic rate measures the speed at which basic, constant processes within the body are taking place and, in particular, how much oxygen a person uses in a given time. A normal male between the ages of 20 and 50 produces 38 to 40 calories of heat every hour for every square meter of body surface, or about 1 calorie per kilogram of body weight. This figure does not vary with height, weight, or general body size in healthy men. The basal metabolism indicates whether or not heat is produced at a greater or smaller rate than is normal for most people in developing energy from food and oxygen.

When a basal metabolism test is made, the person rests after arising in the morning, without having had any breakfast, and breathes from a tank containing a measured amount of air. The rate at which the oxygen in that air is consumed indicates the level of the basal metabolism. A range of 7 plus to 7 minus, relative to the average, is considered normal. Some persons, however, have rates as low as 25 minus without ill-effect on their health. The basal metabolism is also determined by giving radioactive iodine and measuring with a Geiger counter the rate with which the thyroid takes up the iodine. Children who are active and growing have a noticeably higher rate than the average. Various factors cause the basal metabolic rate to be greater than normal. Intense emotions, such as fright or rage, speed up the metabolism, as do certain diseases, such as hyperthyroidism.

Lowered basal metabolism is noted in such bodily states as sleep or undernourishment. It is also found in persons who are anemic, have certain nervous disorders or thyroid deficiency. Inadequacy of either the pituitary or the adrenal gland may have the same effect, while excessive action by either can raise the basal metabolism.

The basal metabolism of a pregnant woman remains at its usual level until the last two or three months before birth. Then the rate in this period will represent the combined metabolism of both mother and child.

In contrast to physical exertion, mental exercise has little effect on the metabolism. According to one authority, half of a salted peanut would provide all the extra calories needed to support a full hour of intense mental concentration.

► Arthritis, Rheumatism, and Gout, *Metabolic Disorders,* 242.

BASEDOW'S DISEASE. *See* EXOPHTHALMIC GOITER; GOITER.

BCG VACCINE. The letters BCG indicate the bacillus first noted by Calmette and Guérin, two researchers of the Pasteur Institute. It is a vaccine used as a means of increasing resistance to tuberculosis, which is spread chiefly from one person who has it to those who have not.

The vaccine is made from a bovine strain of tubercle bacilli, weakened by growth on potato glycerin and bile for several years. The supporters of BCG vaccine point out that it has been successfully used on many millions of children and adults all over the world. *See also* IMMUNIZATION.

BATHING, the total or partial immersion of the body in a medium such as air, vapor, sand, or water, in order to cleanse, soothe, stimulate, heat, cool or irritate it.

Bathing habits of people vary according to their habits and living conditions. The routine use of soap for cleansing is recent. In ancient times, people oiled the skin, and sometimes cleansed themselves with a sweat or Turkish steam bath. Soap cleanses the skin by breaking up or emulsifying the oily secretions and then dissolving them. Thus the layer of grease is removed and the accumulated dirt along with it.

For cleansing the body, a moderately warm bath or shower—from 95° to 100° F.—with soap is best, with thorough washing of portions of the body likely to perspire and acquire odor. Usually the best cleansing soap is ordinary white soap which is easily rubbed into a lather. A soft washcloth helps to cleanse parts of the body difficult to reach. The soap lather should be thoroughly washed from the body with plenty of water since soap left on the skin may irritate it. Brisk rubbing with a towel stimulates circulation and will not injure ordinary skin. However, patting dry with a soft towel is better than rubbing the body if the skin is delicate.

Persons with extremely dry, sensitive, or itching skin may irritate the condition by excessive numbers of hot soapy baths; in many cases, a mild cleansing and oiling is sufficient.

Cool baths conduct heat away from the body and are often recommended to lower the temperature in fever. Hot water causes dilation of the superficial blood vessels and such excess stimulation causes profuse sweating. In taking a hot-water bath, the temperature should be about 98° at the start and then be increased to 115°. Remaining too long in a hot bath may lead to exhaustion and even collapse. A quick cold shower or bath often called a tonic bath, is stimulating because of the sudden change in temperature which produces an immediate contraction of the blood vessels. After the tonic bath, rubbing the body vigorously with a rough towel adds to the stimulation. A cold shower or bath does not agree with many people, and there is no evidence that it is particularly healthful or that it will harden the body against catching colds. *See also* HYGIENE; SKIN.

► The Skin, *Bathing,* 2121.

BATHING BABY. Bath time usually means fun for a baby and warm satisfaction for the mother and father sharing his pleasure. Care and sure handling can help him keep this pleasure. Water too hot or too cold, soap in his eyes, being left unguarded, may make him fear his bath for some time. Sensing uncertainty in an adult can also make him afraid. New mothers and fathers who are hesitant about handling an infant often benefit from infant-care courses like those given by local chapters of the American National Red Cross, Public Health, and Visiting Nurse Associations.

The folding bath-table-and-tub is versatile and convenient, but the baby can be bathed in a large pan or even in the kitchen sink if it is well scoured. Lining the pan or sink with a towel helps prevent slipping and makes the baby more comfortable. Make sure no hot water is left dripping for baby to touch. A shelf or tray within arm's reach of the bath might contain:

Sterilized absorbent cotton in covered container (for extra convenience, cotton balls or a cotton-picker package)
Large rustproof safety pins
Mild pure soap and soap dish
Sterile gauze pads, belly bands, and small bottle of rubbing alcohol for unhealed navel (or antiseptic ointment recommended by doctor)
Paper bag or other receptacle for used cotton

Other articles that should be on hand at bath time are:

Large soft towel for table or bather's lap
Towel for drying
Cotton receiving blanket
Soft washcloth
Baby's clothes

The room in which the baby is bathed should be warm and not drafty, and the water temperature about 90 to 100 degrees. A bath thermometer offers certainty, but the standard test of the water feeling comfortably warm to your elbow or wrist is dependable. Procedure for bathing a baby varies, but the following is a good general outline:

1. With baby wrapped in towel, gently wash face and neck with clear water and dry; after first few months this can be done in bath. The mouth should not be washed. The eyes normally are cleansed by tears; corners may be wiped gently if necessary. Dried mucus or dust at rim of nostrils can be gently wiped with cotton or washcloth; sticks, whether cotton-covered or not, should not be used. Only the outer ears need be washed, with cloth or cotton; dirt or wax in inner ears moves naturally outward, and ears should never be probed.

2. Two or three times a week gently lather head and rinse quickly but thoroughly from the forehead backward. Thorough washing of scalp helps prevent "cradle cap." The "soft spot" or fontanel has a

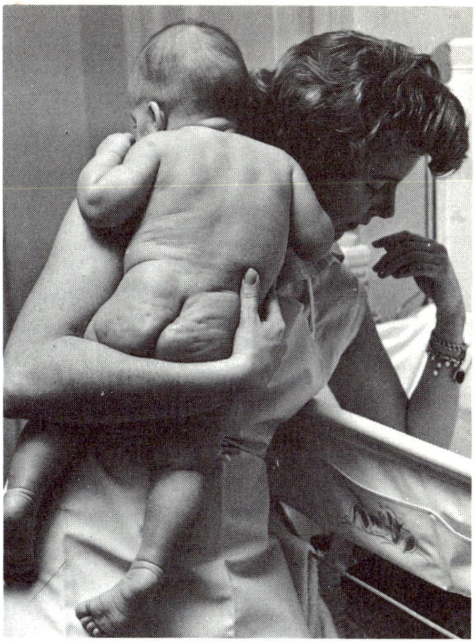

Bathing Baby — With care and sure handling a baby usually enjoys his bath. Soap in his eyes, uncomfortable room or water temperature, or being left unguarded can make him fearful. Water can be tested with the elbow or wrist so that it is not too hot or too cold. The baby should be patted dry. Bath time should be leisurely, and should come before a meal and usually at the same time daily.

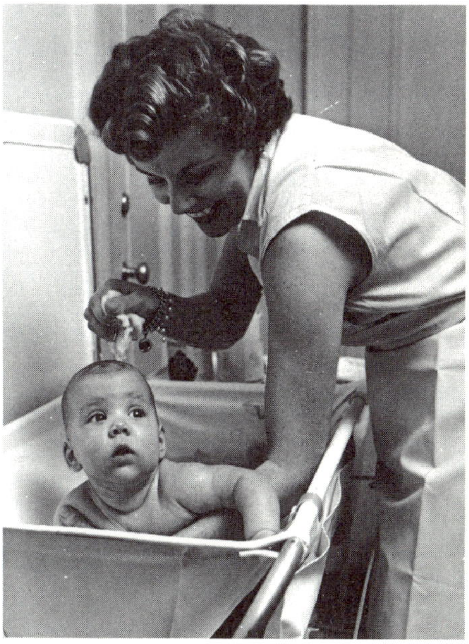

tough covering and is not so easily injured as inexperienced parents fear.

3. Lift baby gently into bath, containing perhaps just a few inches of water to begin with. For a secure grip, place your arm beneath his head, with thumb around his upper arm and fingers under armpit; when he is on his stomach, same grip can be used, with your arm beneath his chest.

4. Soap baby's body thoroughly with your hand or a washcloth. With a girl, separate lips of vulva and wash gently; with a boy (uncircumcised), bring foreskin back as far as it will go easily, and clean tip of penis with cotton, then gently pull foreskin back into place.

5. When baby is thoroughly rinsed, lift him out onto towel on table or your lap; pat him dry (don't rub), with special attention to creases.

Sponge bath: With baby lying on towel on flat surface, follow same general procedure outlined above. Since baby won't be rinsed in a tub, special care must be taken to rinse thoroughly with cloth dipped in clear water; excess soap can irritate the skin.

Oil bath: Under certain conditions, some doctors may recommend that a baby can be given an oil bath and in such cases will give instructions on how to give it.

Most young babies have a bath daily, but your doctor may feel this is unnecessary. It's a good idea to give the bath at the same time of day, however, and before a feeding, not after. But not right before feeding, or you might have a hungry, crying baby on your hands. The most important thing about the time is to allow lots of it. An unhurried, relaxed bath period offers more than good hygiene—the baby can enjoy his natural responsiveness to water, and parents can join in the fun.

► Care and Feeding of the Child, *The Baby's Bath,* 1778.